...agement
Pocket Guide

5th Edition

Dana F. Oakes
Scot N. Jones
Sean P. Shortall

RespiratoryBooks.com

a division of:
Health Educator Publications, Inc.
9220 Lake Carol Drive
Zebulon, North Carolina
United States of America
27597

Copyright © 2022

Oakes' Ventilator Management Pocket Guide
5th edition

ISBN 978-0-932887-49-8

Health Educator Publications, Inc.
Copyright under the Uniform Copyright Convention. All rights reserved. No part of this book may be reproduced, stored in a retrieval system, or transmitted in any form or by any means, electronic, mechanical, photocopying, recording or otherwise, without written permission of the Publisher.

Printed in HONG KONG

RespiratoryBooks
A Division of Health Educator Publications, Inc.
9220 Lake Carol Drive
Zebulon, NC 27597

To order direct: RespiratoryBooks.com

Disclaimer:

The Authors and Publisher have exerted every effort to ensure that the clinical principles, procedures, and practices described herein are based on current knowledge and state-of-the-art information available from acknowledged authorities, texts, and journals. Nevertheless, they cannot be considered absolute and universal recommendations. Each patient situation must be considered individually. The reader is urged to check the package inserts of drugs and disposable equipment and the manufacturer's manual of durable equipment for indications, contraindications, proper usage, warnings, and precautions before use. The Author and Publisher disclaim responsibility for any adverse effects resulting directly or indirectly from information presented in this book, undetected errors, or misunderstandings by the readers.

Author Team

Dana F. Oakes, BA, RRT, RRT-NPS
Educational Consultant/Author

Formerly:
Director of Respiratory Care
V.A. Medical Center
Washington, D.C.

Director of Clinical Education
Respiratory Care Program
Columbia Union College
Tacoma Park, Maryland

Scot N. Jones, BA, RRT, RRT-ACCS
Educational Consultant/Author

Lead Educator
Oakes Academy

Formerly:
Director of Clinical Education
Broward College
Coconut Creek, Florida

Supervisor, Respiratory Care
Vidant Medical Center
Greenville, North Carolina

Sean P. Shortall, RRT, RRT-NPS, RPFT
Senior Respiratory Therapist
Pulmonary Diagnostics Lab
Northern Light Eastern Maine Medical Center
Bangor, Maine

Assistant Editors

As is always the case, producing a new edition is a dynamic, synergistic process. The final product is a testimony to the efforts of an exceptional team of professionals.

Lori Badgley, MSRC, RRT
Lab Coordinator/Adjunct Faculty
Lincoln Land Community College
Springfield, Illinois

Respiratory Therapist
Memorial Medical Center
Springfield, Illinois, USA

Joseph Buhain, EdD, MBA, RRT, FAARC
Formerly:
Program Director for Respiratory Therapy and Simulation
Saint Paul College
Saint Paul, Minnesota

Clinical Patient Training Program Manager
Patient Services, Respiratory Health
Hill-Rom, Inc.
Shoreview, Minnesota

United States Naval Medical Officer (Reserve)
Prior United States Combat Army Medic
Minneapolis, Minnesota

Lexie Caraway, MBA, RRT, RRT-ACCS, RRT-NPS, AE-C
Manager of Respiratory Therapy
Sarah Bush Lincoln Health Center
Mattoon, Illinois

Edwin L. Coombs, Jr., MA, RRT, RRT-NPS, RRT-ACCS, CPFT, FAARC
Senior Director of Marketing, Portfolio Training, Clinical Affairs, & Intensive Care
Draeger, Inc.
Telford, Pennsylvania

Gracielle Fong, MSHE, RRT, RRT-NPS
Assistant Professor
Director of Clinical Education
Respiratory Therapy Program
County College of Morris
Randolph, New Jersey

Deborah Ketchen, RRT
Respiratory Therapist
Pen Bay Medical Center
Rockport, Maine, USA

Dewayne Kibble, RRT
Respiratory Therapist
Signature Healthcare of Cleveland
Cleveland, Tennessee

Lauren McAvoy, BS, RRT, RRT-NPS, RRT-ACCS
Respiratory Therapist

Angela Reid, MRC, RRT, RRT-ACCS
ACCS Respiratory Therapist
Mercy Health Hospital
Youngstown, Ohio, USA

Assistant Professor, Clinical Adjunct
Youngstown State University
Austintown, Ohio, USA

Keith Siegel, MBA, RRT, CPFT, FAARC
President/Owner
Siegel Respiratory Consulting, Inc.
Union, Maine

Executive Director
U.S. COPD Coalition
Union, Maine

Danielle Schryver, MSc, RRT
Respiratory Therapy Program Director
Kennebec Valley Community College
Fairfield, Maine

Lee E. Wisdom, MHS, RRT, RRT-ACCS, RRT-NPS
Registered Respiratory Therapist
Norton Audubon Hospital
Louisville, Kentucky

CONTENTS
detailed contents on following pages

Initial Considerations	1
Parameters/Operation	2
Modes	3
Assessment	4
Graphics	5
Equations	6
Clinical Management	7
Noninvasive Ventilation	8
Diseases/Disorders	9
Ventilator Effects	10
Weaning	11
Appendix	A
Index	

TABLE OF CONTENTS

1 Initial Considerations
Ventilator Support
  Indications 1-2
  Contraindications 1-3
Acute Respiratory Failure
  Types of 1-4
  Causes of (Differential Checklist) 1-5
Clinical Parameters 1-8
Objectives of Mechanical Ventilation 1-9
Ventilator Initiation Checklist 1-10

2 Types and Parameters
Types of Ventilation
  Full vs Partial 2-2
  Pressure vs Volume 2-3
Parameters
  Overview 2-4
  Volumes 2-5
  Pressures 2-8
  Others 2-15
Operating Relationships
  Volume 2-24
  Pressure 2-27
  Oxygenation 2-28

3 Modes of Ventilation
Mode Classification 3-2
Breath Types 3-2
Mode Chart 3-3
Modes (key) 3-4
Volume
  Volume A/C 3-6
  Volume SIMV 3-8
  Volume MMV 3-10

Pressure
- Pressure A/C 3-12
- Pressure SIMV 3-14
- Pressure Support 3-16
- Pressure MMV 3-18
- APRV/BiVent/Bilevel 3-20

Pressure Ventilation with a Target
- Volume Assured Pressure Support (VAPS) 3-26
- Pressure Regulated Volume Control (PRVC) 3-29
- Adaptive Pressure Ventilation (APV) 3-31
- Proportional Assist Ventilation (PAV) 3-32
- Proportional Pressure Support (PPS) 3-32
- SmartCare/PS 3-34
- Volume Support (VS) 3-35
- Adaptive Support Ventilation (ASV) 3-37

Other Modes and Adjuncts
- Continuous Positive Airway Pressure (CPAP) 3-38
- Automatic Tube Compensation (ATC) 3-39
- Automode 3-40
- Neurally-Adjusted Ventilatory Assist (NAVA) 3-41
- Extracorporeal Membrane Oxygenation (ECMO) 3-51
- High-Frequency Oscillatory Ventilation (HFOV) 3-54

4 Assessment
Assessing Respiratory Distress 4-2
- Troubleshooting the Patient 4-4
- Troubleshooting the Ventilator 4-5

Patient-Ventilator Assessment
- Considerations for Patient Assessment 4-6
- Considerations for Ventilator Assessment 4-7
- Acid-Base Values 4-9
- Oxygenation 4-10
- Ventilation 4-11
- Ventilation Mechanics 4-12
  - Static Compliance (Cstat) 4-13
  - Dynamic Compliance (Cdyn) 4-13
  - Airway Resistance (Raw) 4-14

Troubleshooting
See also Graphics Chapter
- Changes in V$_T$ 4-16
- Changes in Rate 4-17

Changes in PIP	4-18
Changes in PEEP	4-19
Other Troubleshooting	4-20
Asynchrony	4-21

5 Ventilator Graphics

Explanations/Introduction 5-3
Types of Graphics
  Scalars
    Pressure-Time 5-4
    Volume-Time 5-7
    Flow-Time 5-9
  Loops
    Pressure-Volume 5-11
    Flow-Volume 5-14
Normal Graphics
  Scalars 5-16
  Loops 5-22
Abnormal Graphics
(by waveform)
  Scalars 5-26
  Loops 5-30
(by problem)
  Patient
    Air-Trapping (auto-PEEP) 5-36
    Airway Resistance Changes 5-38
    Compliance Changes 5-41
    Active Exhalation 5-43
    Partial Obstruction 5-44
  Ventilator
    Overdistension 5-45
    Leaks 5-46
    Rate (Cycle) Asynchrony 5-48
    Flow Asynchrony (Flow Starvation) 5-49
    Trigger Asynchrony 5-50
Other Applications 5-52

6 Equations

- Acid-Base 6-2
- Oxygenation 6-4
- Ventilation 6-12
- Ventilator Calculations
  - General 6-16
  - Weaning 6-17
  - Mechanics 6-19
- Hemodynamic Monitoring 6-23
- Patient Calculations 6-29
  - IBW and PBW 6-29
  - Gas Duration 6-30

7 Clinical Management

- Airway Management
  - Bag-Valve-Mask 7-2
  - Airway Adjuncts 7-3
  - Endotracheal Tubes 7-4
    - Intubation 7-5
  - Tracheostomy Tubes 7-8
- Ventilation Management
  - Improving 7-15
  - Acute Respiratory Acidosis 7-16
  - Acute Respiratory Alkalosis 7-18
  - Metabolic Disorders 7-19
  - Permissive Hypercapnia 7-20
- Oxygenation Management
  - Improving 7-21
  - Estimates 7-21
  - Strategies for Improving 7-22
  - PEEP 7-24
- Airway Clearance Management
  - Suctioning 7-37
  - Other Methods 7-39
- Humidity Management
  - Overview 7-42
- Patient/Ventilator Synchrony
  - Artificial Airway 7-45
  - Auto-PEEP 7-45
  - Expiratory Valves 7-46
  - Humidifier 7-46
  - Trigger Sensitivity 7-47

Mode Asynchrony	7-49
Flow Asynchrony	7-50
Cycle Asynchrony	7-50

8 Noninvasive Ventilation
Types
High-Flow Oxygen Therapy	8-2
CPAP	8-3
NPPV (BiPAP)	8-4
Acute Respiratory Failure (Management)	8-8
Contraindication	8-9
Interfaces	8-10
Management Considerations	8-11
Monitoring for Success	8-12
Discontinuing	8-12

9 Diseases/Disorders
ARDS	9-2
Asthma	9-11
Bariatrics	9-16
Bronchopleural Fistula	9-18
Burns (Thermal, Smoke Inhalation)	9-20
Cardiac, Acute (MI, CHF)	9-22
Cardiac, Postoperative	9-24
COPD Exacerbations	9-25
COVID (see Viral Pulmonary Disorders)	
Drug Overdose	9-29
Guillain-Barre Syndrome (see Neuromuscular)	
Lung Abscess (see Unilateral Disorders)	
Lung Transplantation (see Unilateral Disorders)	
Myasthenia Gravis (see Neuromuscular)	
Neuromuscular Disorders	9-31
Pneumonia (see Unilateral Disorders)	
Poisoning (see Drug Overdose)	
Postoperative Care	9-33
Restrictive Disorders	9-34
Trauma (Chest)	9-35
Trauma (Head)	9-38
Unilateral Disorders	9-42
Independent Lung Ventilation	9-43
Viral Pulmonary Disorders (COVID, etc.)	9-44

10 Ventilator Effects

Pulmonary
- Airway Obstruction 10-2
- Atelectasis/Derecruitment 10-3
- Auto-PEEP (Air Trapping) 10-4
- Hyperoxic Lung Injury (Toxicity) 10-8
- Respiratory Drive (Decreased) 10-9
- Ventilation/Perfusion Imbalance 10-10
- Work of Breathing 10-11
- Lung Injury 10-12
- Hypoventilation 10-14
- Hyperventilation 10-15

Extrapulmonary
- Cardiac 10-16
- Neurological 10-16
- Nutritional 10-17
- Hepatic 10-17
- Gastrointestinal 10-17
- Renal 10-17

Ventilator-Associated Infections
- Ventilator-Associated Events 10-19
- VAE/VAP Bundle 10-20

11 Weaning

- Weaning/Discontinuation Algorithm 11-2
- Basic Definitions 11-4
- General Strategies 11-5
- Assessment for Weaning/Discontinuation 11-6
  - Vital Signs 11-6
  - Oxygenation 11-7
  - Ventilation 11-7
  - Mechanics 11-8
  - Integrated Indices 11-8
  - Acid-Base Balance 11-9
  - Airway 11-10
  - Chest Imaging 11-11
  - Ventilator Muscle/Strength 11-11
  - Ventilator Drive/Demand 11-11
  - Cardiovascular 11-12
  - Electrolytes 11-13

Metabolic	11-13
Nutritional	11-13
Neurological	11-14
Pharmacological	11-15
Renal	11-15
Psychological	11-16
Miscellaneous	11-17
Procedural	11-17
Summarized Indications of Failure	11-18
Rapid Shallow Breathing Index (RSBI)	11-19
Cuff Leak Test	11-20
Extubation Procedure	11-21
Post-Extubation Care	11-22
Reintubation Criteria	11-23
Weaning and Discontinuation Summarized Guidelines	11-24

A   Appendix

Basic Units of Measure	A-2
Gas Phase Symbols	A-2
Blood Phase Symbols	A-2
Conversions	
Metric	A-3
U.S./Metric Equivalents	A-3
Temperature (C ↔ F)	A-4
Weight (kg ↔ lb)	A-4
Height (ft ↔ in ↔ cm)	A-4
Abbreviations	A-5
Evidence-Based Guidelines (AARC)	A-7

Index

Terminology and Notations
A few basic terms are listed here because they are foundational for the book (used frequently!). We made a decision to spell out abbreviations wherever practical, but other abbreviations can be found in the appendix.

Invasive Mechanical Ventilation: Providing (usually positive) pressure ventilation by either an endotracheal tube or tracheostomy tube.

Noninvasive Ventilation (NIV): Providing (usually positive) pressure ventilation without an endotracheal or tracheostomy tube. This is usually by some form of a face mask or nasal prongs.

We have chosen to use **NPPV** (noninvasive positive pressure ventilation) for what many clinicians refer to as BiPAP (which is a branded name). CPAP (continuous positive airway pressure) remains as CPAP (not a branded name).

Negative Pressure Ventilation: this is normal physiologic respiration and can be mimicked with mechanical ventilation (Cuirass, "Iron Lung" are examples) but is clinically rare. A negative pressure is created within the pulmonary system, creating a "negative" gradient compared to ambient pressure (at the mouth or stoma).

Positive Pressure Ventilation: The reverse of physiologic ventilation, where a positive pressure is created at the mouth/stoma. The great majority of invasive and noninvasive mechanical ventilation uses positive pressure ventilation.

Subscripts: In most places we have gone with a modified subscript notification (O_2 instead of O_2) for readability in the pocket guide.

Units: We have listed units for measures, unless we felt leaving them off left no confusion (and actually clarified the layout for use at the bedside).

> Any use of brand names in this pocket guide is meant to be illustrative or to clarify using bedside terminology. This is not meant as an endorsement of any product or manufacturer.

Adult versus Neonatal/Pediatric Ventilator Management

This pocket guide is intended for adult ventilator management (unless otherwise specified). While the basic principles (assessment, modes, graphics, etc.) can certainly be applied to neonatal/pediatric patients, specific recommendations may not apply appropriately.

See Oakes' Neonatal/Pediatric Respiratory Care Pocket Guide (RespiratoryBooks.com) for detailed noninvasive and invasive ventilatory strategies.

1 INITIAL CONSIDERATIONS

Ventilator Support
    Indications 1-2
    Contraindications 1-3
Acute Respiratory Failure
    Types of... 1-4
    Causes of (Differential Checklist) 1-5
Clinical Parameters 1-8
Objectives of Mechanical Ventilation 1-9
Ventilator Initiation Checklist 1-10

INDICATIONS

Assumptions

- Unless specifically noted, considerations are for invasive ventilatory support (see noninvasive chapter or diseases/disorders for specifics related to noninvasive management)

- Because applying negative pressure ventilation is uncommon, considerations apply to positive pressure ventilation.

- Every patient must be considered individually. There is a complex relationship that exists between a patient's acute process and their underlying overall well-being, comorbidities, age, etc.

Indications for Ventilatory Support

Indications	Description	Clinical Examples
Apnea	Absence of breathing	• Cardiac Arrest
Acute Respiratory Failure (ARF)	Inability to maintain adequate oxygenation (PO_2) and/or ventilation (PCO_2)	• Hypoxemic respiratory failure • Hypercapnic respiratory failure See pg 1-4
Impending Respiratory Failure	Respiratory failure is imminent despite reasonable interventions. *Commonly defined as:* Patient is minimally maintaining (or gradual deterioration of) normal acid-base but with significant WOB.	• Worsening clinical parameters (vitals, ABGs, labs, etc.) with • Evidence of distress/tiring (work of breathing, level of consciousness, etc.)
Chronic Respiratory Failure	Repeated failures after attempts to liberate from the ventilator (weaning trials, extubation attempts, etc.)	• Significant respiratory weakening (COPD, pulmonary fibrosis)
Prophylactic Ventilatory Support	Clinical indication = high risk of respiratory failure. Ventilatory support is instituted to ↓ WOB, minimize O_2 consumption and hypoxemia, reduce cardiopulmonary stress, and/or control airway with sedation.	• Head injury • Heart muscle injury • Major surgery • Shock (prolonged) • Burns/Smoke injury • Trauma

Contraindications to Invasive Ventilatory Support

Absolute Contraindications

- Advanced directives (do-not-intubate)
  Consider discussion of DNI (for example, if anticipated short need for ventilation for surgery) or other palliative options (NIV, for example)

- Untreated tension pneumothorax
  Stabilize the pneumothorax emergently, then place on positive pressure ventilation

Relative Contraindications/Considerations

- Other less invasive therapies have potential for success
  Consider the indications for noninvasive ventilation (see chapter 8). If goals can be met noninvasively, they likely should be (decreases potential for infection, morbidity, and mortality)

- Determination of inability to wean
  Some severe diseases (end-stage) may indicate the need for invasive ventilation, but the overall prognosis for weaning is poor. A discussion should occur with the patient/family and clinical team prior to intubation, when possible.

Two Types of Acute Respiratory Failure

	Hypoxemic Respiratory Failure	Hypercapnic Respiratory Failure
Terminology	Type I Acute Respiratory Failure	Type II Acute Respiratory Failure
Definition	The failure of lungs /heart to provide adequate O_2 for metabolic needs	The failure of the lungs to eliminate adequate CO_2
Criteria	(at sea level)* $PaO_2 < 60$ mmHg on $FiO_2 \geq 0.50$ or $PaO_2 < 40$ mmHg on any FiO_2 $SaO_2 < 90\%$ CO_2 is normal/low	Acute ↑ in $PaCO_2 > 50$ mmHg or Acutely above normal baseline in COPD with concurrent ↓ in pH < 7.30
Select Causes	• Right-to-left shunt • V/Q insufficiencies/mismatching (severe pneumonia, pulmonary edema, ARDS, sepsis, etc.) • Alveolar hypoventilation • Diffusion defect (at A/C membrane) Usually results in refractory hypoxemia (increasing FiO_2 doesn't increase PaO_2 as much as expected)	• Decreased respiratory drive (sedatives, stroke, sleep apneas, obesity hypoventilation, metabolic alkalosis, hypothermia) • Decreased neuromuscular/thoracic function (chest wall, spinal injury, muscle disorders, drugs) • Increased dead space (PE, dynamic hyperinflation, hypoventilation) • Increased CO_2 production (fever, sepsis, overnutrition, metabolic acidosis)

*Values will vary slightly at higher altitudes, including during air transport

Acute Respiratory Failure:
A Differential Checklist

Pulmonary	
Acute Airway Obstruction	• Anaphylaxis • Aspiration • Bleeding (airway) • Bronchoconstriction • Edema/inflammation (including epiglottitis) • Foreign objects • Secretions • Smoke/chemicals • Tracheal/bronchial malacia or stenosis
Asthma, COPD	• Exacerbation • Severe
Decreased Lung Tissue Functioning (Severe)	• ARDS • Atelectasis • Fibrosis • Pneumonia • Pulmonary edema • Pulmonary embolism (PE)
Sleep Disordered Breathing	• Obstructive sleep apnea (OSA)
Chest Wall	
Chest Wall	• Flail chest • Kyphoscoliosis / Scoliosis (Severe)/Kyphosis (Severe), pectus deformities (carinatum, excavatum) • Obesity • Rib fracture • Severe burns
Intrathoracic	
Intrathorax	• Empyema • Hemothorax • Pleural Disease/Effusions • Pneumothorax

Initial Considerations

CNS Depression	
CNS	• Cerebral Ischemia, CVA • Drug misuse/overdose: alcohol, anesthetics, barbiturates, cocaine/heroin, methadone, morphine, sedatives, narcotics, etc. • ↑ ICP (hypoxic brain) • Infection • Lesions/tumors • Metabolic alkalosis (CSF) • Obesity hypoventilation (Pickwickian) • Primary hypoventilation (Ondine's Curse) • Sleep apnea (central) • Trauma

Neuromuscular	
Neuro-muscular	• Amyotropic Lateral Sclerosis (ALS) • Pharmacology: antibiotics, Ca^{++} channel blockers, anticholinesterase, curare/non-depolarizers, dexamethonium, methyl alcohol, nerve gases, succinylcholine • Electrolyte imbalance • Guillian-Barré syndrome, myasthenia gravis • High spinal injury/disease • Multiple sclerosis • Muscular dystrophy • Myotonia • Phrenic nerve injury • Poisons/toxins: botulism, mushrooms, paraquat, petroleum distillates • Poliomyelitis, polymyositis • Rabies, SLE, status epilepticus, tetanus

Cardiovascular	
Cardio-vascular	• Cardiac arrest (↓ CO) • CHF with pulmonary edema • Congenital heart disease • Hypovolemia • Shock • Thromboemboli (cardiac)

Other	
Other	• Anxiety • Hypothyroidism • Malnutrition/fatigue • Mechanical ventilation (air-trapping) • Metabolic acidosis • Post-operative complications

Clinical Parameters to Consider in Determining Need

Parameter*	Normal	Support Indicated
Ventilation		
$PaCO_2$	35-45 mmHg	50-55 mmHg or acute ↑ from pt. baseline
pH	7.35-7.45	< 7.25
V_D/V_T	25-40%	> 60%
Oxygenation		
PaO_2	80-100 mmHg (Room Air)	< 50 mmHg (Room Air) < 60 mmHg (50% O_2) < 200 mmHg (100% O_2)
SaO_2	> 95%	< 75%
$P(A-a)O_2$	10-25 mmHg (Room Air)	< 350 mmHg on 100% O_2
PaO_2/F_IO_2	350-400 mmHg	< 200 mmHg
Mechanical Capabilities (Mechanics)		
V_T (ideal)	5-8 mL/kg	< 5 mL/kg
f	12-20 bpm	< 10 or > 35 prolonged
$\dot{V}_E$	5-6 L/min	> 10 L/min
VC (ideal)	60-75 mL/kg	< 15 mL/kg
FEV_1 (ideal)	50-60 mL/kg	< 10 mL/kg
FRC	60% or higher	< 50% predicted
P_I max (MIP, NIF)	more negative than -60 to -80 cmH_2O	more positive than -20-30
Respiratory pattern	Normal	Abnormal/Irregular

*Values vary by study, and may vary individually based upon gender and age

Initial Considerations

Objectives of Mechanical Ventilation*

Consider these objectives while providing support. Ask, "what objectives of support are being targeted?" and "Are the objectives being satisfactorily addressed with this treatment?"

Physiological Objectives

- **Support or Manipulate Pulmonary Gas Exchange**

    Alveolar Ventilation = pH directly, $PaCO_2$ indirectly
    Goal is an acceptable pH (not always a normal pH)

    Arterial Oxygenation = PaO_2, SaO_2, CaO_2, SpO_2
    Achieve acceptable level using acceptable F_IO_2.
    In most cases, $SaO_2 > 90\%$ or $PaO_2 > 60$ mmHg

- **Decrease the Risk of Ventilator-Related Lung Injury**
    Goal may include using acceptable values (pH, $PaCO_2$, PaO_2) instead of normal values in order to protect the lungs

Clinical Objectives

- Provide support when airway patency needs to be established (invasive)
- Reverse hypoxemia/hypoxia
- Reverse acute respiratory acidosis
- Relieve respiratory distress
- Prevent or reverse atelectasis
- Reverse ventilatory muscle fatigue (unload ventilatory muscles)
- Permit sedation and/or neuromuscular blockade
- Decrease systemic or myocardial oxygen consumption
- Stabilize the chest wall

*Adapted in part from ACCP Consensus Conference:
Mechanical Ventilation; **Respiratory Care**, Vol. 38, #12, 1993.

Initial Considerations

Ventilator Initiation Checklist

Right Ventilator	• Choose ventilator by setting (short-term/PACU, critical care, transport, etc.) • Ensure proper circuit attached (single-limb vs dual-limb, adult vs pediatric/neo) • Ensure appropriate filters to protect patient and equipment • Ensure "red" outlet used when available (connects to generator during power loss) • Perform pre-use/circuit check (leak, battery, alarms, etc.) before initiation (even if urgently needed)
Right Mode	(see modes, chapter 3) • Ensure a mode that provides sufficient support for clinical situation • Ensure a mode that allows for optimized synchrony
Right Settings	(see parameters, chapter 2) • Ensure that generic settings (those used clinically most often) are titrated to meet patient's clinical needs
Right Alarms	(see alarms, chapter 2) • Ensure alarms are set safely (not too wide, not too narrow) • Ensure alarms that act as limits (often high pressure alarm) are set carefully to allow for adequate ventilation but not risk patient harm
Assess	Once initiated, confirm all ventilator settings using clinical context: ventilator graphics, mechanics (PIP, Pplat), etc. Reassess after induction drug wears off.

RSI: Rapid Sequence Intubation

2 TYPES and PARAMETERS

Types of Ventilation
    Full vs Partial 2-2
    Pressure vs Volume 2-3
Parameters
    Overview 2-4
    Volumes 2-5
    Pressures 2-8
    Others 2-15
Operating Relationships
    Volume 2-24
    Pressure 2-27
    Oxygenation 2-28

Clinical Notes

- Set parameters vary by mode of ventilation chosen (see chapter 3)
- While generic/starting parameters are usually used, each parameter for each patient should be evaluated for optimization, avoiding hazards related to each. This is the art of ventilator management.

Types of Mechanical Ventilation

	Full	Partial
Definition	Ventilator does all the work of breathing necessary to maintain effective alveolar ventilation.	Patient and ventilator share the WOB necessary to maintain effective alveolar ventilation.
Goals	Achieves **total control** of the patient's ventilatory pattern – patient does not trigger or assist	Achieves only **partial control** of the patient's ventilatory pattern – allows the patient to breathe either spontaneously or trigger (assist) the ventilator.
Indications	• Need to decrease O_2 consumption (respiratory failure, cardiac failure) • Underlying disease process (neuromuscular) • Pharmacologic therapy (deep sedation, paralysis)	• Maintains respiratory muscle tone • Encourages vent-patient synchrony • Weaning/discontinuation (spontaneous breathing trials, etc.)
Clinical Notes	• There's a clinical difference between locking a patient out (not allowing spontaneous contributions, such as with traditional CMV) and aiming for full vent support to address indications • Full support may quickly lead to muscle wasting or atrophy	The actual amount of support provided varies by mode (see mode chapter) and parameter settings (trigger, etc.)
Example Modes	• Traditional CMV Modes • Modes with "high" settings leading to a higher than patient-driven minute ventilation, excessive trigger, etc.	• Assist-Control • SIMV • Pressure Support • Volume Support • Dual Level (APRV, etc.)

SIMV: Synchronized Intermittent Mandatory Ventilation

Volume vs. Pressure Ventilation

Ventilators, in general, either primarily manipulate volumes or pressures to provide ventilatory support. It is important to remember that when you manipulate one, the other is affected. Note that research is inconsistent in whether there is a true "best" type of ventilation.

	Volume Ventilation	**Pressure Ventilation**
Terms	Volume-limited Volume-targeted Volume-controlled Volume-cycled	Pressure-limited Pressure-targeted Pressure-controlled
Key	Volume is set (constant) Pressure varies (you can control the tidal volume, but inspiratory pressures may vary)	Pressure is set (constant) Volume varies (you can control the inspiratory pressure, but tidal volumes may vary)
Definition	The ventilator ends inspiration after a **set volume** is reached	The ventilator ends inspiration after a **set inspiratory pressure is delivered for a specific amount of time (set time) or at a set flow**
Advantages	A set volume is delivered, unaffected by changes in compliance, resistance Allows for more precise manipulation of $PaCO_2$	Limits risk of pressure injury (barotrauma) Some pressure modes (PRVC, APV) allow for targeted V_T while keeping pressure-targeting as a priority
Disadvantages	Increased risk of alveolar over-distension (PIP and Pplat)	Tidal volumes (and minute ventilation) may be inconsistent

Types and Parameters

Parameters

Conventional Ventilator Parameters Overview

Noninvasive parameters are addressed more completely in the Noninvasive chapter

Some parameters (such as those associated with HFOV, APRV, etc.) are listed within the specific mode - see Modes chapter

Parameter	Average Normal Values
Volumes	
Minute Ventilation ($\dot{V}E$)	5-10 L/min
Tidal Volume (V_T)	~6 mL/kg IBW *(lung protection)* 6-8 mL/kg IBW *(typical)*
Pressures	
Peak Inspiratory Pressure (PIP)	15-25 cmH$_2$O
Mean Airway Pressure (mPAW)	5-15 cmH$_2$O
Positive End Expiratory Pressure (PEEP)	4-7 cmH$_2$O
Other	
Frequency (*f*) or Rate	12-20 breaths/min
I:E Ratio	1:2 to 1:3
Inspiratory Time (T_I)	~0.9 - 1.2 sec
Flow Waveform	Decelerating, Square, Sinusoidal
O$_2$% (F$_I$O$_2$ if decimal)	21% - 100% (< 50% when possible)

Ventilator Volumes

Minute Ventilation ($\dot{V}_E$, MV) the amount (volume measured in liters) of air moved in and out of the lungs in 1 minute	
Average Range	5-10 L/min
Clinical Notes	$\dot{V}_E = f \times V_T$ (assumes no effort) Use an average of several tidal volumes Use an average of several tidal volumes With Spontaneous Modes: Minute ventilation is calculated by averaging return tidal volumes by total rate. With a mix of spontaneous/vent breaths: $\dot{V}_E =$ [SET f x Set V_T (or return V_T)] + [Spont f x Spont V_T] Insufficient $\dot{V}_E$: hypoventilation, possible hypoxemia Excessive $\dot{V}_E$: hyperventilation, injury Minute ventilation is not usually set directly (MMV being the exception - see pg 3-10 and 3-18) but is a critical value to monitor. It can be an indicator of underlying issues (metabolic acidosis, fever, etc.). A clinically appropriate $\dot{V}_E$ is one that ensures an adequate pH and $PaCO_2$ in context of disease or disorder.

Tidal Volume (VT)	
the volume of air delivered to (or exhaled from) the lungs with each breath	
Average Range	• 6-8 mL/kg IBW for lung protection • 6-10 mL/kg IBW for normal lungs (> 8 mL/kg IBW is unusual clinically)
Clinical Notes	*In the absence of VT measurement, aim for a gentle rise and fall of the chest.* • Set in volume ventilation, may be set as a target in some pressure modes • In pressure-controlled modes, VT is an indicator of changing lung dynamics (compliance, resistance) • In pressure-controlled modes, set inspiratory pressure is usually titrated to ensure a safe tidal volume range (see Usual Range, above) • Once tidal volume is set within a safe range, it is generally maintained there unless plateau pressures indicate the need to decrease
Cautions	• Most clinicians favor a tidal volume in the lower part of the appropriate range to avoid volutrauma. There are exceptions to this (such as neuromuscular disorders). • There are differences between ideal body weight (IBW) and predicted body weight (PBW), both of which have been used in evidence-base (see next page) • A tidal volume too large may lead to volutrauma and barotrauma (indirectly) • A tidal volume set too low (< 4 mL/kg IBW) may lead to ineffective alveolar ventilation

Calculating Tidal Volumes
See notes on IBW vs. PBW in Clinical Notes, below

Step 1: Determine PBW (or IBW)*
    PBW: Predicted Body Weight
    IBW: Ideal Body Weight

PBW (female) kg = 45.5 + [0.91 x (Height in cm - 152.4)]
PBW (male) kg = 50 + [0.91 x (Height in cm - 152.4)]

IBW (female) kg = 45.5 + [0.9 x (Height in cm - 154)]
IBW (male) kg = 50 + [0.9 x (Height in cm - 154)]

Step 2: Multiply PBW (or IBW) by desired mL/kg (usually 6-8)

PBW (kg) x desired mL/kg = calculated tidal volume
IBW (kg) x desired mL/kg = calculated tidal volume

Alternative Option (a Bedside Method)

1. Calculate Ideal Body Weight in Pounds (lbs)
   IBW (female) lb = 100 + 5 x (Height in inches - 60)
   IBW (male) lb = 106 + 6 x (Height in inches - 60)

2. Convert Pounds (lbs) to Kilograms (kg)
   IBW (kg) = IBW (lb) / 2.2

3. Multiply IBW (kg) by desired mL/kg (usually 6-8)

Clinical Notes
- **The best practice is to measure height, then record in the medical record. Estimating height risks inaccurate set or targeted tidal volumes.**
- PBW vs. IBW: ARDSnet is technically based upon PBW, even though IBW is often used clinically. Note that the calculations are quite close. IBW results in a clinical underestimation of V_T compared to PBW:

    In a 5-ft-5-in female, PBW is 57-kg, IBW is 55.4-kg
    Setting a V_T of 8 mL/kg: PBW 456 mL, IBW 443 mL

Ventilator Pressures

see following pages for details

Parameter	Set	Not Set
PIP	in pressure modes	in volume modes
PEEP	X	
mPAW		X
Pplat		X
Driving pressure		X

Pressures Graphical Representation

(shape and measures vary based on mode, parameters, and patient characteristics)

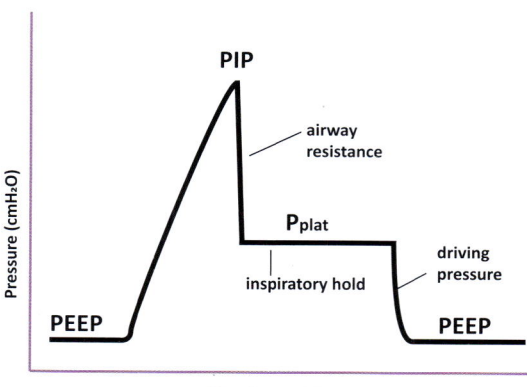

2-8 Types and Parameters

Peak Inspiratory Pressure (PIP, IP, P$_{peak}$)
Highest (peak) proximal airway pressure reached during inspiration

Average Range	15-25 cmH$_2$O (above PEEP) maintain < 30 cmH$_2$O (lung injury prevention) titrate PIP to deliver a V$_T$ (see V$_T$ for details)
Clinical Notes	The lowest PIP that adequately ventilates the patient is usually appropriate IP (PIP) is set in pressure-control ventilation. Increasing PIP increases V$_T$ (and mPAW) Decreasing PIP decreases V$_T$ (and mPAW)

	Increased	Decreased
Compliance	V$_T$ increases	V$_T$ decreases
Resistance	V$_T$ decreases	V$_T$ increases

	With a set PIP, increasing T$_I$ will increase V$_T$ When high PIPs are used to open collapsed alveoli, the open alveoli may over-distend, resulting in volutrauma
Cautions	PIP doesn't distribute evenly throughout the lungs. Pressure will follow the "path of least resistance" which has a tendency to overly distribute to higher compliance areas, which are potentially the healthier units. Rapidly changing (increasing) C and FRC places the patient at high risk for lung over-distension and resultant air leaks. V$_T$ should be continuously monitored. Set low $\dot{V}_E$ and low V$_T$ alarm carefully PIP too low: atelectasis, hypoventilation PIP too high: barotrauma, hemo compromise
Selecting Initial PIP	PIP is set in pressure modes: V$_T$ = PIP - PEEP 1. Adjust PIP to a target tidal volume range 2. Use the Pressure-Volume Loop: adjust PIP until there is little/no flattening of the loop

Positive End Expiratory Pressure (PEEP)
pressure maintained at the end of each exhalation through some type of impedance

Ranges	3-5 cmH$_2$O is minimal to maintain FRC (5 is commonly used initially) Higher PEEP is used therapeutically (maintain open-lung approach without causing hemodynamic compromise)
Types	**Intrinsic PEEP** (air-trapping, auto-PEEP, dynamic hyperinflation) is PEEP caused by disease/disorder (COPD, etc.) or inappropriate settings (inadequate expiratory time) **Extrinsic PEEP** (set PEEP) is a vent parameter used either physiologically (to offset loss of PEEP when the vocal cords are bypassed) or therapeutically. Measured with an expiratory hold. **Total PEEP** = Intrinsic + Extrinsic
Clinical Notes	PEEP is used to prevent airway/alveolar collapse and establish functional residual capacity (FRC). Primarily used to improve oxygenation (↑ FRC), but recruited lung units may improve V/Q, thus improving ventilation secondarily Excessive PEEP: over distension of alveoli, which may lead to air-trapping, decreased venous return to the heart, and increased PVR Inadequate PEEP: atelectasis (especially in areas of lower compliance)

Optimal PEEP	Optimal PEEP is the optimization of oxygenation with the goal of preventing end-expiratory atelectasis while not causing alveolar over-distention (and hemodynamic compromise)
	Techniques:
	see page 7-26 for more details
	1. Incremental PEEP (increase PEEP, monitor change in VT with close watch of hemodynamics)
	2. PEEP/FiO_2 tables (ARDSnet)
	3. Use P-V loop (approximately 2-3 cmH₂O above the lower inflection point) to set PEEP, allow for recruitment, and then wean using P-V loop. Preferred: Use the ventilator's tool, when available, for setting PEEP.
	4. Oxygenation PEEP Study
	5. Esophageal Pressure
Monitoring	Increase in PaO_2
	CXR: monitor under/over expansion
	P-V Loop: shift of PIP down at same VT (VT should be set)

Types and Parameters

Mean Airway Pressure (mPAW, MAP, PA̅W)	
average (mean) proximal airway pressure through the entire respiratory cycle	
Average Range	5-15 cmH$_2$O
Clinical Notes	**mPAW** is often the most critical factor in determining optimal oxygenation as it correlates with lung volume. Generally, there is a linear rise in mean PaO$_2$ with ↑ mPAW until over-distension occurs, then a ↓ PaO$_2$ (and ↑ PaCO$_2$) occurs. *Factors affecting mPAW (in probable order of magnitude):* PEEP, TI, PIP/VT, f (↓TE), V̇I, and pressure waveform (see diagram below) **Approximation of mPAW:** $$mPAW = \frac{\left[\frac{(PIP \times T_I)}{Total\ Cycle\ Time} + (PEEP \times T_E)\right]}{Total\ Cycle\ Time}$$ *Optimal level:* The lowest level in which gas exchange is most efficient and beyond which alveolar over-distension occurs

Methods to Improve mPAW

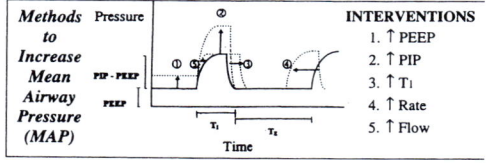

Plateau Pressure (P$_{plat}$, P$_{alv}$)	
average (mean) alveolar pressure during inspiratory phase	
Average Range	maintain < 30 cmH$_2$O for lung protection
Clinical Notes	Technically is the pressure applied to both the small airways and alveoli The higher the Pplat, the greater the risk of barotrauma. Has to be measured during peak inspiration, during a time when there is no air movement in the lungs This is completed by performing an inspiratory hold/pause (usually a button that needs to be pushed) for 0.5-1.0 second, although some sources recommend 3+ seconds (shorter holds may overestimate Pplat) Look at pressure scalar during maneuver to show a defined plateau (waviness in plateau may suggest inaccuracy) Used as a determinant of static compliance and airway resistance Some clinical situations may result in an inaccurate (false high) Pplat, including external chest wall pressure (pregnancy, obesity, etc.) and spontaneous respiratory effort during the maneuver.

Types and Parameters

Driving Pressure (ΔP, DP)	
A calculation that indicates the pressure above PEEP applied to the the entire respiratory system to achieve a tidal volume	
Average Range	14-18 cmH$_2$O may be considered safe*
	> 15 cmH$_2$O (or an increase of 7+) indicates potential for lung injury and increased mortality
Clinical Notes	**Calculating ΔP**
	ΔP = Pplat - PEEP
	Sources vary on defining a safe or target driving pressure
	Interpretation of driving pressure may be more sensitive to lung injury than Pplat alone (acceptable VT with Pplat < 30 may still result in a high driving pressure)
	ΔP is a combination of both lung expansion and chest wall expansion so either can influence it.
	May be inaccurate in presence of air trapping (overestimates driving pressure)

* Williams E, Motta-Ribeiro G, Vidal Melo M. Driving pressure and transpulmonary pressure: How do we guide safe mechanical ventilation? Anesthesiology 2019;131(1):155-163.

Other Parameters

Frequency (*f*) or Rate	
quantity of breaths over a minute	
Average Range	12-20/minute
Clinical Notes	There are really several types of rates, depending on the mode being used: **Set Rate:** Rate of breaths delivered by the ventilator (*f*) **Spontaneous Rate:** The rate of the patient independent of the ventilator (RR) Manipulating the rate is used to manipulate the $PaCO_2$ and pH (increase rate to decrease $PaCO_2$, which will increase pH) **Calculating a New Rate Based on $PaCO_2$** New Rate = $\dfrac{\text{Current Rate} \times \text{Current PaCO}_2}{\text{Desired PaCO}_2}$ • For disorders requiring lower VT (such as ARDS), higher *f* may be required to maintain an adequate $\dot{V}_E$. • For obstructive disorders, a lower *f* may be required to allow for sufficient expiratory time (to avoid or relieve air trapping), sometimes as much as allowing for an overall I:E ratio of 1:6.
Cautions	High rates decrease available expiratory time and may lead to air-trapping with inadvertent PEEP, which risks a ↓ venous return and ↓ cardiac output.

Inspiratory Time (TI)	
duration of the inspiratory phase	
Average Range	0.9-1.2 seconds (set to an appropriate I:E ratio)
Clinical Notes	Select TI for patient comfort and synchronous breathing. Considerations include lung time constants, patient age, and breathing pattern. | ↓ C | Short TC | Use short TI | | ↑ Raw | Long TC | Use long TI | TC = Time Constant
Cautions	The longer the TI (especially > 1.0 sec) the greater the risk of barotrauma, adverse cardiac effects. Carefully observe flow waveforms to ensure exhalation to baseline (see flow-time scalar and flow-volume loop on pg 5-37) Longer TI = ↓ TE (assuming same rate) Changing TI in pressure modes will change the tidal volume (the amount of time at a set pressure being increased or decreased)

Inspiratory pause:

Once common in clinical practice, the inspiratory pause is a delay in the onset of expiration after inspiration (flow ceases). It was utilized as a tool of oxygenation and aerosol dispersion, but has fallen out of favor due to lack of favorable evidence of benefit to oxygenation, an increase in asynchrony, etc.

Inspiratory Flow ($\dot{V}_I$)	
the rate at which gas is delivered to the patient during the inspiratory phase	
Average Range	40-100 L/min
Clinical Notes	**Volume Ventilation** (if able to set): set to lowest value that will generate the desired PIP/Pressure waveform Minimum flow should be ~ 2-3x the minute ventilation Higher flows may be needed to maintain V_T when T_I is shortened, and may decrease WOB in patients with high inspiratory demand Slower $\dot{V}_I$s are used for patients with ↑ Raw and/or poor gas distribution (to ↓ PIP and risk of barotrauma) **Pressure Ventilation**: Flow is determined by patient characteristics
Cautions	**Signs of insufficient flow:** Desired PIP not reached with mandatory breaths ↑ WOB (retractions, etc.) Pressure fluctuations on manometer around baseline PEEP setting Ventilator asynchrony Graphics: displays a characteristic "figure eight" (as patient's demand outstrips delivered flow pressure decreases while volume increases)

Flow Waveform	
Most Common	Decelerating waveforms are generally preferred
Clinical Notes	Decelerating Square Sinusoidal

Types and Parameters

Inspiratory:Expiratory Ratio (I:E Ratio)	
ratio of inspiratory time to expiratory time	
Average Range	1:2 to 1:3
Clinical Notes	I:E Ratio is usually not set directly. Setting the RR and TI (or Flow Rate) determines the I:E Ratio. $PaCO_2$ is seldom altered significantly by altering I:E Ratio. Altering PIP and PEEP is usually more effective. I:E ratios with a longer expiratory time may be indicated with obstructive disorders (COPD, asthma, etc.) to avoid auto-PEEP I:E ratios with a lesser expiratory time are cautiously considered for patients needing an increased mPAW (ARDS, etc.)
Cautions	Inverse ratios carry a high risk of auto-PEEP and the potential for hyperinflation, barotrauma, ↓ CO, and cerebral injury

Expiratory Time (TE)	
time duration of the expiratory phase of a breath	
Clinical Notes	TE is usually not set, but is the result of the rate and TI
	Calculating Expiratory Time
	TE = $(60/f)$ - TI
Cautions	Care should be taken to observe expiratory time, which can best be assessed by observing the flow volume loop or scalar, ensuring that exhalation returns to baseline before the next breath begins

Expiratory Hold (end-expiratory pause)	
delay in the onset of inspiration with the prevention of any further exhalation (just before inspiration)	
Clinical Notes	Maneuver used to measure auto-PEEP (assuming no spontaneous efforts during the maneuver) May be manually performed by holding designated expiratory-hold button/function for 3-5 sec (allows alveolar pressure to equilibrate, flow needs to be ~0) In some ventilators, auto-PEEP has to be calculated by subtracting the extrinsic PEEP (that which is set) from the total PEEP (that which is measured in this maneuver)

Types and Parameters

FiO₂
Fraction of Inspired Oxygen (FiO₂) -- decimal equivalent

Oxygen Percentage (O₂ %)

these terms are nearly interchangeable (and commonly expressed as a percentage value even when referred to as FiO₂)

Average Range	0.21 - 1.0 (or 21% - 100% as a percentage) (maintain < 0.50 whenever possible)
Clinical Notes	FiO_2 increases alveolar O_2 (PAO_2) which, assuming sufficient physiology, increases arterial O_2 (PaO_2)

Calculating a New FiO₂ Based on PaO₂
New $FiO_2 = \dfrac{\text{Desired } PaO_2 \times \text{Current } FiO_2}{\text{Current } PaO_2}$

Insufficient O_2 (hypoxemia) may lead to tissue hypoxia and potentially death, so should be carefully avoided

Administering supplemental oxygen (especially in moderate-to-high amounts) has risks (free radicals, increased inflammatory response, cell damage, etc.). Careful consideration for maintaining minimum (not necessarily normal) Oxygen thresholds are usually preferred.

Inspiratory Trigger *(Sensitivity)*	
the level of spontaneous effort (flow, pressure, or neural signal) needed to trigger the ventilator to move into the inspiratory phase.	
Average	Flow is most common: set to allow for effective triggering without causing auto-triggering (no effort that triggers a breath)
Clinical Notes	Flow triggers are most common clinically and use minimal work of breathing.
	Pressure triggers require more effort and may increase work of breathing, some of which may be insurmountable for the patient. May be necessary with strong cardiogenic oscillations (a bounding heartbeat that triggers the ventilator)
	Neural triggers require a special endotracheal tube (see NAVA on page 3-41), but when set correctly may help facilitate more natural triggering of the ventilator.
	Too sensitive: will result in auto-cycling that triggers breaths without patient or rate input (asynchrony)
	Not sensitive enough: results in "locking" the patient out where a breath can't be initiated when wanted (asynchrony)

Expiratory Trigger (Sensitivity):
This is found in pressure support ventilation, defined as the percentage of peak inspiratory flow (as patient flow slows) at which the ventilator cycles from inspiration to expiration.

Humidification

the goal of humidity is to replace the humidity lost when bypassing the upper airway (caused by an artificial airway) or when flows are beyond what the body can physiologically keep up with (such as with high flow therapies)

Types	**HME (Heat and Moisture Exchanger)** in general, collects the patient's heat and humidity on expiration, then passes it back to the patient on inspiration. Active HME: A specially designed HME in which either heat and/or humidity are added **Active humidity** typically uses a heated passover humidifier (other types exist, including wick humidifiers, ultrasonic, etc.). Maintained around body temperature or slightly below.
Clinical Considerations	Consider transitioning from an HME to active humidity when*: • Thick and/or copious secretions • Loss of VT (leak in patient or cuff) • Low VT strategies (ARDS) • Hypothermic patients (Temp < 32° C) • High minute ventilation (> 10 L/min)

* *Summarized from Restrepo, R, Walsh, B. AARC: CPG: Humidification During Invasive and Noninvasive Mechanical Ventilation. Respir Care 2012;57(5):782-788.*

Ventilator Alarms

Some ventilator require properly set alarms to function properly: high pressure alarm as a limit, for example

Initial Settings	Alarm	Setting
	Apnea	< 20 sec
	High/Low $\dot{V}_E$	10-15% +/- set $\dot{V}_E$
	High/Low V_T	10-15% +/- set V_T
	High/Low PIP	10 cmH$_2$0 +/- avg. PIP
	High/Low PEEP	3-5 cmH$_2$0 +/- set PEEP
	High/Low F$_I$O$_2$	5% +/- set F$_I$O$_2$
	High/Low Rate	10-15 /min +/- set rate
	I:E Ratio	when I>E
	Temp	2° above/below set temp.

Typical Problems:

Problem	Consequence
Alarms too sensitive	Results in alarms that activate too often, resulting in alarm fatigue. Alarm fatigue occurs when hospital staff become desensitized to alarms and may become less likely to respond to a legitimate alarm event
Alarms set too wide (not sensitive enough)	Unaware of changing clinical condition, including tiring/distress

Types and Parameters

Volume Ventilation: Operating Relationships

Further explanation on next page

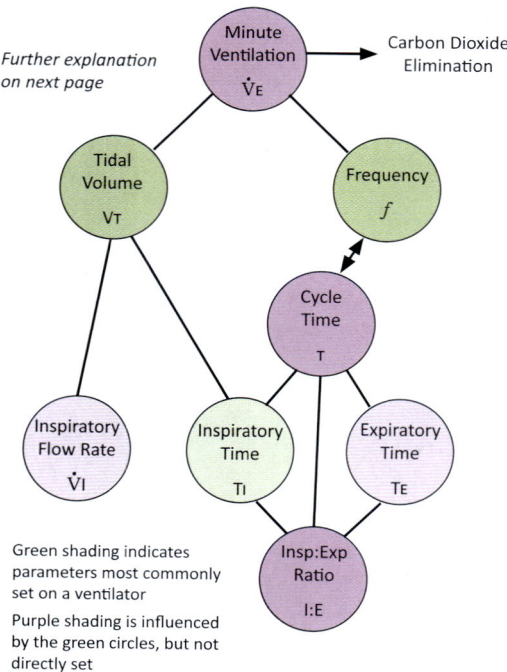

Green shading indicates parameters most commonly set on a ventilator

Purple shading is influenced by the green circles, but not directly set

Adapted from Chatburn, R.L. and Lough, M.D.: Mechanical Ventilation. In Lough, M.D. et al: *Pediatric Respiratory Therapy*, copyright 1985 by Mosby Yearbook.

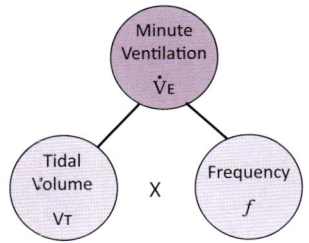

Minute Ventilation

$$\dot{V}_E = V_T \times f$$

Clinically, minute ventilation is usually manipulated by altering f, leaving V_T alone

---

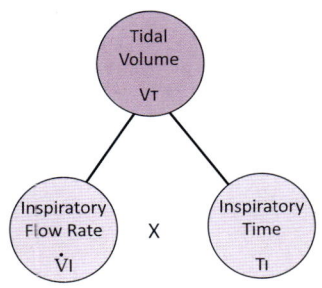

Tidal Volume

$$V_T = \dot{V}_I \times T_I$$

Types and Parameters

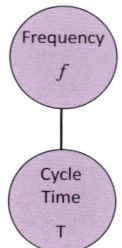

Frequency/ Cycle Time

$T = 60 / f$
$f = 60 / T$

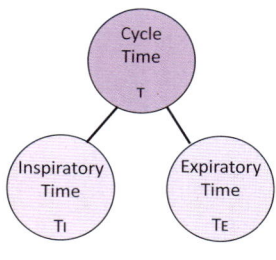

Cycle Time

$T = T_I + T_E$

Cycle time is the combined inspiratory (usually active) + expiratory (usually passive) times.

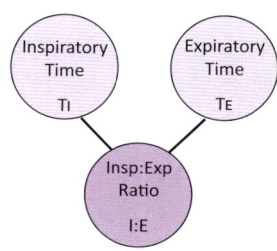

I:E Ratio

$$I:E = \frac{1}{(T_E/T_I)}$$

Understanding the I:E ratio is critical, particularly in ensuring an adequate expiratory time (enough time to empty the lungs)

Pressure Ventilation: Operating Relationships

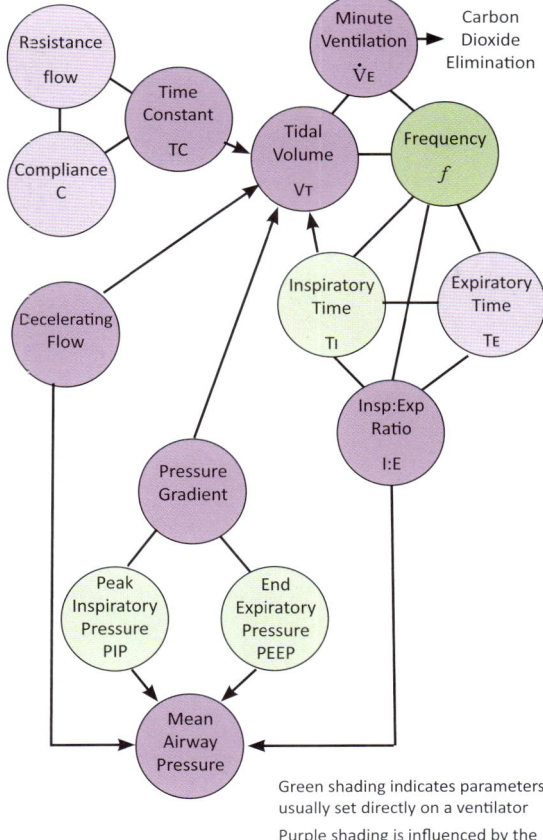

Green shading indicates parameters usually set directly on a ventilator

Purple shading is influenced by the green circles, but not directly set

Types and Parameters

Oxygenation Determinants

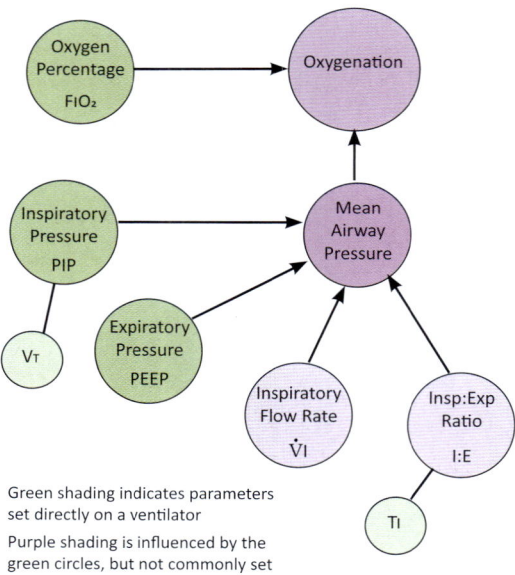

Green shading indicates parameters set directly on a ventilator

Purple shading is influenced by the green circles, but not commonly set

Adapted from Carlo, W.A., Greenough, A. Chatburn, R.L.: Advances in mechanical ventilation. In Boynton B.R., Carlo W.A., Jobe A.H. [Eds.]: ***New Therapies for Neonatal Respiratory Failure: A Physiologic Approach***. Cambridge, Cambridge University Press, 1994, p. 134

3 MODES OF VENTILATION

Mode Classification 3-2
Breath Types 3-2
Mode Chart 3-3
Modes (key) 3-4

Selecting a Mode

A selection of modes are covered in this chapter. This is not meant to be comprehensive but a guide to navigating through basic princ ples.

In general, evidence has not supported any one mode being superior to another. The best mode is the mode best managed, with careful consideration for patient synchrony, lung protection, and other clinical goals (recruitment, acid-base balance, etc.), within the context of current evidence-base and available equipment.

Mode Classification

Modes focus primarily on manipulation of inspiration. Exhalation, as with normal physiology, is usually passive (HFOV is an exception)

How Inspiration:	Initiates	Sustains	Terminates
This is called the breath's:	Trigger	Limit	Cycle
It can be controlled by:	Patient		
	Pressure Flow Neural	Pressure Volume Flow Neural	Pressure Volume Flow Neural
	Ventilator		
	Time (Rate)	Pressure Volume Flow	Pressure Volume Flow Time (Ti)

Breath Types

Breaths	Inspiratory Phase Variables		
	Trigger	Limit	Cycle
Ventilator-Cycled Breaths			
Ventilator (control) breath	Vent	Vent	Vent
Assisted breath	Patient	Vent	Vent
Patient-Cycled breath:			
Supported breath	Patient	Vent	Patient
Spontaneous breath	Patient	Patient	Patient

Modes

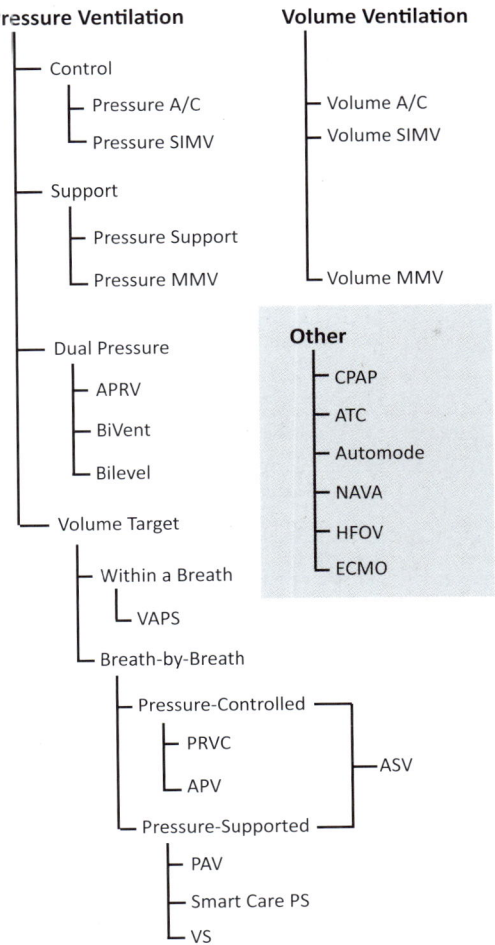

Modes 3-3

Mode (and Page) Key

Use this list with the previous page.

Volume Ventilation		Page
V-A/C	Volume Assist/Control Ventilation	3-6
V-SIMV	Volume Synchronized Intermittent Mandatory Ventilation	3-8
V-MMV	Volume Mandatory Minute Ventilation	3-10
Pressure Ventilation		
P-ACV	Pressure Assist/Control Ventilation	3-12
P-SIMV	Pressure Synchronized Intermittent Mandatory Ventilation	3-14
PSV	Pressure Support Ventilation	3-16
P-MMV	Pressure Mandatory Minute Ventilation	3-18
APRV	Airway Pressure Release Ventilation	3-20
BiVent	(see APRV)	
Bilevel	(see APRV)	
Pressure Ventilation with a Target Volume		
VAPS	Volume Assured Pressure Support	3-26
PRVC	Pressure Regulated Volume Control	3-29
APV	Adaptive Pressure Ventilation	3-31
PAV / PPS	Proportional Assist Ventilation / Proportional Pressure Support	3-32
SmartCare/PS	SmartCare Pressure Support	3-34
VS	Volume Support	3-35
ASV	Adaptive Support Ventilation	3-37

Modes

Other Modes and Adjuncts		Page
CPAP	Continuous Positive Airway Pressure	3-38
ATC	Automatic Tube Compensation	3-39
Automode		3-40
NAVA	Neurally-Adjusted Ventilatory Assist	3-41
ECMO	Extracorporeal Membrane Oxygenation	3-51
HFOV	High-Frequency Oscillatory Ventilation	3-54

1. Modes (names, classifications, etc.) can be very confusing, in part due to manufacturers' reluctance to standardize terminology. What follows in this chapter is a simplified, quick reference approach to the current modes.
2. Many of these modes lack evidence-based support, making the best choice of mode that which the Respiratory Therapists and Physicians have the most expertise with in the context of the specific patient clinical situation.
3. Volume ventilation can also be called volume-controlled, -cycled, -limited or -targeted ventilation.
4. Flow-limited or flow-controlled is synonymous with volume-limited or volume-controlled.
5. Closed-Loop Ventilation refers to modes that auto-titrate (somehow) in response to changing patient condition. Examples include NAVA, ASV, and Automode (see each for more details)

Initial Settings with Specific Modes:

- Typical **Initial Settings** for parameters like V_T, PIP, T_I, etc., can be found in detail in Chapter 2.
- **Disease-specific recommendations** (including mode selection where appropriate) can be found in Chapter 10.

Modes

Volume - Assist/Control (V-A/C)	
Summary	• A combination of assisted and/or controlled (mandatory) ventilation • All breaths are delivered at a set V_T and $\dot{V}_I$ • In between the controlled (set rate) breaths, a patient can trigger a full machine (assisted) breath at the same parameters as the controlled breath (i.e., V_T and $\dot{V}_I$). Note that pure "controlled" ventilation (CMV) also exists which does not allow for patient triggering (this locks the patient out).

	Classified By:		
Breath Type	**Trigger**	**Limit**	**Cycle**
Assisted	Patient (flow or pressure)	Vent (flow or volume)	Vent (volume)
Controlled	Vent (time = rate)	Vent (flow or volume)	Vent (volume)

Indications
- Full to partial ventilatory support is appropriate for patients receiving heavy sedation/paralysis, drug overdose, spinal cord or head injury with no (or minimal) respiratory drive
- Provides maximum amount of "rest" (only real work of breathing is triggering the vent if drive to breathe is present), assuming settings have been optimized

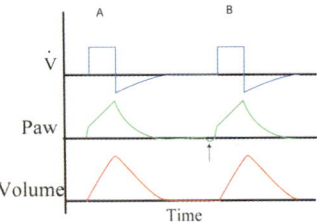

A: Time-triggered (vent) = Controlled breath
B: Patient-Triggered (see arrow) = Assisted breath

Note that volume is equal in both breaths

Clinical Notes

- Guarantees a tidal volume and minimum minute ventilation (Pt can trigger additional vent breaths, increasing minute ventilation)
- Barotrauma is a risk (set high pressure limit carefully)
- Flow is fixed (may cause asynchrony if higher flow or volume demand)
- May cause or worsen air trapping (dynamic hyperinflation)
- Over time may result in respiratory muscle atrophy
- Patients with a high RR (due to head injury, for example) may over-trigger breaths, resulting in a respiratory alkalosis

Volume - Synchronized Intermittent Mandatory Ventilation (V-SIMV)	
Summary	A combination of spontaneous and mandatory ventilation • The ventilator will deliver a set number of mandatory (controlled) breaths per minute. • These mandatory breaths will be at a preset V_T and $\dot{V}_I$ • The patient may breathe spontaneously in between the mandatory machine breaths from the baseline pressure. The breath may be assisted with pressure support. • If the patient begins to inspire just prior to the time-triggered mandatory (control) breath, a full vent-assisted breath will be delivered. Pressure-supported breaths may ↑ patient comfort, while controlled breaths (with longer T_I) ensure mPAW and lung recruitment

	Classified By:		
Breath Type	**Trigger**	**Limit**	**Cycle**
Assisted	Patient (flow or pressure)	Vent (flow or volume)	Vent (volume)
Controlled	Vent (time = rate)	Vent (flow or volume)	Vent (volume)
Spontaneous	Patient (flow or volume)	Vent (pressure)	Patient (pressure or flow)

Indications
- Full to partial ventilatory support is appropriate for patients receiving heavy sedation/paralysis, drug overdose, spinal cord or head injury with no (or minimal) respiratory drive
- Some clinicians use SIMV as a method to wean patients (decreasing the set rate increases spontaneous breaths)

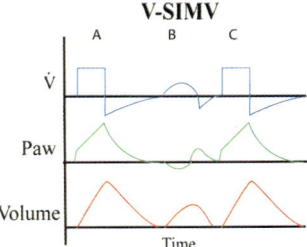

A: Controlled + Time triggered
B: Spontaneous breath (no pressure support)
C: is synchronized and assisted
Breaths A + C are both full ventilator (volume) breaths

Clinical Notes:
- Guarantees a set number of tidal volume breaths, ensuring a minimum minute ventilation
- May maintain respiratory muscle strength (avoids atrophy)
- There is coordination between spontaneous and mandatory breaths
- Spontaneous breaths may be pressure supported (see PSV)
- Spontaneous breathing may produce better gas distribution and less cardiac output compromise
- High pressure limit must be set appropriately to minimize the risk of alveolar injury
- Patient WOB may increase if flow rate/sensitivity are not set correctly
- Possible tachypnea with fatigue and hypercapnia if mandatory (control) rate is set too low (inadequate ventilatory support or weaning too rapidly) or if pressure support for spontaneous breaths is inadequate
- Some evidence suggests SIMV weaning may result in longer weaning times

*Hess D. Ventilator modes used in weaning. **Chest** 2001; 120:6 Supp. 474S-476S

Volume - Mandatory Minute Ventilation
(V-MMV)

Summary	This is a form of spontaneous ventilation but with a guaranteed (set) minute ventilation. It is a form of closed loop ventilation where the ventilator makes changes independently after predicting the patient's ability to meet or exceed the set minute ventilation.
	• Spontaneous breaths are the baseline
	• A minimum minute ventilation is set (usually 70-90% of current minute ventilation)
	• The ability to meet the set minute ventilation is analyzed by the ventilator: the average of a set number of breaths, the average of a set period of time, etc. (depends on the ventilator)
	• If the minute ventilation is unlikely to be met with spontaneous breaths, some help is provided by the ventilator (giving set V_T breaths in the case of V-MMV) until the minimum minute ventilation is achieved.

	Classified By:		
Breath Type	**Trigger**	**Limit**	**Cycle**
Assisted	Patient (flow or pressure)	Vent (flow or volume)	Vent (volume)
Controlled	Vent (time = rate)	Vent (flow or volume)	Vent (volume)
Spontaneous	Patient (flow or pressure)	Vent (pressure)	Patient (pressure or flow)

Indications
- Primarily neonates, infants, pediatric patients who are spontaneously breathing and determined to be ready to wean
- May be appropriate for patients with an unstable ventilatory drive

Clinical Notes
- When possible, calculate IBW and determine appropriate baseline minute volume needed prior to initiation
- Minute ventilation ($\dot{V}_E$) may not provide adequate alveolar ventilation ($\dot{V}_A$) with rapid, shallow breathing. Ensure an appropriate high rate alarm.
- PIPs are variable, increasing barotrauma risk
- An inadequate set $\dot{V}_E$ (less than spontaneous $\dot{V}_E$) can lead to inadequate support and patient fatigue
- An excessive set $\dot{V}_E$ (greater than spontaneous $\dot{V}_E$) with no spontaneous breathing can lead to total support

Pressure - Assist/Control
(P-A/C)

Summary	<ul><li>A combination of assisted and/or controlled (mandatory) ventilation</li><li>All breaths are delivered at a set IP and TI</li><li>In between the controlled (set rate) breaths, a patient can trigger a full machine (assisted) breath at the same parameters as the controlled breath (i.e., PIP and TI).</li></ul>Note that pure "controlled" ventilation (CMV) also exists which does not allow for patient triggering (this locks the patient out).

Caution: Some ventilators (and some versions of the same ventilator) set Pressure Control (PIP) relative to the set PEEP, while in others the set Pressure Control is the "true" PIP (above baseline). Sometimes this is also referred to as **PEEP-compensated or **not-PEEP-compensated**.

For example: On one ventilator, a setting of 15/5 results in a PIP of 15 and on another ventilator it is a PIP of 20 (15+5)

	Classified By:		
Breath Type	**Trigger**	**Limit**	**Cycle**
Assisted	Patient (flow or pressure)	Vent (pressure)	Vent (time = TI)
Controlled	Vent (time = rate)	Vent (pressure)	Vent (time = TI)

Indications
- Full to partial ventilatory support is appropriate for patients receiving heavy sedation/paralysis, drug overdose, spinal cord or head injury with no (or minimal) respiratory drive

P-ACV

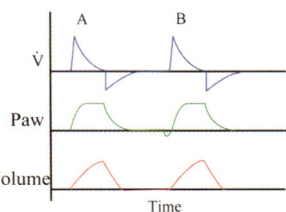

A: controlled and time-triggered
B: is assisted and patient-triggered
Each breath is a full machine pressure breath

Clinical Notes
- Peak pressures are controlled (= no guaranteed V_T)
- Minimal patient WOB (if parameters are properly adjusted)
- Variable inspiratory flow may be more comfortable
- Delivers volume early in the breath (decelerating flow) which may improve gas distribution
- Increased WOB if flow rate/trigger are not set correctly
- Low exhaled V_T and $\dot{V}_E$ alarms must be set properly
- Possible alveolar hyperventilation and possible respiratory alkalosis due to: Inappropriate sensitivity setting (auto-cycling) and/or rapid breathing rate
- May cause or worsen air trapping (dynamic hyperinflation)
- Potential respiratory muscle atrophy (vent is offloading the majority of the work of the respiratory muscles)

Pressure - Synchronized Intermittent Mandatory Ventilation
(P-SIMV)

Summary	A combination of spontaneous and mandatory ventilation
	• The ventilator will deliver a set number of mandatory (controlled) breaths per minute.
	• These mandatory breaths will be at a preset inspiratory pressure (IP) and inspiratory time (TI)
	• The patient may breathe spontaneously in between the mandatory machine breaths from the baseline pressure. The breath may be assisted with pressure support.
	• If the patient begins to inspire just prior to the time-triggered mandatory (control) breath, a full vent-assisted breath will be delivered.
	Pressure-supported breaths may ↑ patient comfort, while controlled breaths (with longer TI) ensure mPAW and lung recruitment

****Caution:** Some ventilators (and some versions of the same ventilator) set Pressure Control (PIP) relative to the set PEEP, while in others the set Pressure Control is the "true" PIP (above baseline). Sometimes this is also referred to as **PEEP-compensated** or **not-PEEP-compensated**.

	Classified By:		
Breath Type	**Trigger**	**Limit**	**Cycle**
Assisted	Patient (flow or pressure)	Vent (pressure)	Vent (time = TI)
Controlled	Vent (time = rate)	Vent (pressure)	Vent (time = TI)
Spontaneous	Patient (flow or volume)	Vent (pressure)	Patient (pressure or flow)

Modes

P-SIMV

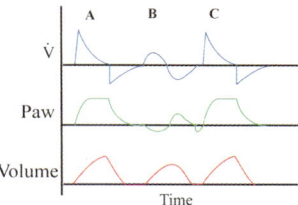

A: controlled and time-triggered
B: spontaneous breath (no pressure support)
C: synchronized and assisted
A and C are full ventilator pressure breaths

Indications
- Full to partial ventilatory support is appropriate for patients receiving heavy sedation/paralysis, drug overdose, spinal cord or head injury with no (or minimal) respiratory drive
- Some clinicians use SIMV as a method to wean patients (decreasing the set rate increases spontaneous breaths)

Clinical Notes:
- Guarantees a set number of breaths, each pressure-limited
- May maintain respiratory muscle strength (avoids atrophy)
- There is coordination between spontaneous and mandatory breaths
- Spontaneous breaths may be pressure supported (see PSV)
- Spontaneous breathing may produce better gas distribution and less cardiac output compromise
- Patient WOB may increase if flow rate/sensitivity are not set correctly
- Possible tachypnea with fatigue and hypercapnia if mandatory (control) rate is set too low (inadequate ventilatory support or weaning too rapidly) or if pressure support for spontaneous breaths is inadequate
- SIMV weaning may result in longer weaning times

*Hess D. Ventilator modes used in weaning. **Chest** 2001; 120:6 Supp. 474S-476S

Pressure Support Ventilation
(PSV)

Summary	A spontaneous mode where the patient triggers all breaths, which are then supported by the ventilator (a set pressure is added to the spontaneous breath)

	Classified By:		
Breath Type	**Trigger**	**Limit**	**Cycle**
Supported	Patient (flow or pressure)	Vent (pressure)	Patient (flow*)

*Pressure supported breaths are flow-cycled: as inspiratory flow slows, the ventilator reads this as the patient being ready to start exhalation, but may be pressure-cycled or time-cycled as a back-up measure on some ventilators.

Operation
- A pressure support (PS) level is set by the clinician, usually not less than 10 cmH$_2$O (ΔP 5+). This may be titrated to a desired V$_T$, but the clinician should remain aware that because pressure is set, V$_T$ will vary with changes in compliance, resistance, and patient effort
- The inspiratory phase ends when the inspiratory flow rate reaches a set minimum flow rate or percentage of the patient's peak flow (ventilator specific). Some newer ventilators have variable cycling criteria known as "expiratory sensitivity" and "inspiratory cycle off". There are also pressure and time cycling criteria as back up measures available on some ventilators.

Indications
- Spontaneously breathing patient who requires support to help overcome work of breathing (compliance or airway resistance) or respiratory muscles weakness
- Spontaneous breathing trials (SBTs = weaning)

PSV

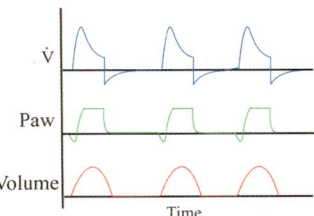

Clinical Notes

- PS, when set correctly, supports the spontaneous tidal volume and may help decrease overall respiratory rate
- PS, when set correctly, supports work of breathing by compensating for resistance related to artificial airways, circuits, etc.
- Patient has greater control over tidal volume, rate, inspiratory time, and inspiratory flowrates
- Note that PS may be used as an independent mode (fully spontaneous) or combined with modes that have spontaneous breaths (SIMV, for example)
- May help facilitate weaning
- It is critical that adequate backup ventilation is set (in case of tiring, apnea) and alarms are appropriate
- PS too low: fatigue and tachypnea are likely. Look for signs of distress (vital signs, accessory muscles, etc.)
- PS too high: increased risk of air-trapping. Try decreasing PS level. If VT, RR are same, consider leaving at lower PS.

Pressure - Mandatory Minute Ventilation
(P-MMV)

Summary	This is a form of spontaneous ventilation but with a guaranteed (set) minute ventilation. It is a form of closed loop ventilation where the ventilator makes changes independently after predicting the patient's ability to meet or exceed the set minute ventilation. • Spontaneous breaths are the baseline • A minimum minute ventilation is set (usually 70-90% of current minute ventilation) • The ability to meet the set minute ventilation is analyzed by the ventilator: the average of a set number of breaths, the average of a set period of time, etc. (depends on the ventilator) • If the minute ventilation is unlikely to be met with spontaneous breaths, some help is provided by the ventilator (giving set pressure breaths in the case of P-MMV) until the minimum minute ventilation is achieved.

	Classified By:		
Breath Type	**Trigger**	**Limit**	**Cycle**
Assisted	Patient (flow or pressure)	Vent (flow or volume)	Vent (volume)
Controlled	Vent (time = rate)	Vent (pressure)	Vent (time = Ti)
Spontaneous	Patient (flow or volume)	Vent (pressure)	Patient (pressure or flow)

Indications
- Primarily neonates, infants, pediatric patients who are spontaneously breathing and determined to be ready to wean
- May be appropriate for patients with an unstable ventilatory drive

Clinical Notes
- Minute ventilation ($\dot{V}_E$) may not provide adequate alveolar ventilation ($\dot{V}_A$) with rapid, shallow breathing. Ensure an appropriate high rate alarm.
- Tidal volumes are variable
- An inadequate set $\dot{V}_E$ (less than spontaneous $\dot{V}_E$) can lead to inadequate support and patient fatigue
- An excessive set $\dot{V}_E$ (greater than spontaneous $\dot{V}_E$) with no spontaneous breathing can lead to total support

Airway Pressure Release Ventilation
(APRV, TCAV, BiVent, BiLevel, Biphasic)

Summary	In essence, this is CPAP (think oxygenation) with releases of pressure (think CO_2 elimination) with a goal of recruitment.
	1. A longer high level (CPAP phase) which allows for alveolar recruitment. The goal is enough pressure to open the lungs, but not so much as to overdistend them.
	2. A very short low level (release phase) which does not allow for full exhalation, "defending" the FRC. The purpose of the low level, also called "the release" is to allow for CO_2 elimination.
	The patient can breathe spontaneously during the high level (APRV), or during both high and low level (BiVent)
	Current clinical thought is that there are 2 uses for APRV:
	1. Rescue (TCAV = Time-Controlled Adaptive Ventilation), spontaneous breathing isn't necessary. See next page.
	2. Recruitment (non-rescue), with an emphasis on using CPAP to recruit, spontaneous breathing is available on top of the CPAP level. See pg 3-22

Note that we have gone with the most common terminology, but this does vary some between manufacturers

	Classified By:		
Breath Type	**Trigger**	**Limit**	**Cycle**
Spontaneous*	Patient (flow or pressure)	Ventilator (pressure)	Patient (flow)
Ventilator	Ventilator (time)	Ventilator (pressure)	Ventilator (time)

*Spontaneous breaths may occur during the ventilator "breaths"

APRV TCAV (Rescue) Initial Suggested Settings

P$_{high}$ **PEEP**$_{high}$ (high pressure level)	20-30 cmH$_2$O (or 2-3 above Pplat) The lower the patient's P/F ratio (or increase the OI), the higher the initial setting needed Match the Pplat if transitioning from another mode (if pressure mode, use PIP)
T$_{high}$ (time spent at high pressure level)	Match the rate from conventional mode (rescue) Rate = (60/current rate) - T low Typically ~ 1-4 seconds (lower if > severe) Thigh is set ~4-6 sec when used purely for recruitment (not rescue)
P$_{low}$ **PEEP**$_{low}$ (low pressure level)	0 cmH$_2$O Allows for maximum ΔP for unimpeded expiratory flow. Setting above zero may add expiratory resistance, inhibiting CO$_2$ removal (the lungs are kept open using Tlow, not Plow)
T$_{low}$ (time spent at low pressure level)	The actual value is less important than using ventilator graphics Typically ~0.2-0.6 seconds (75% of PEF) *Use flow scalar or loop to set expiratory flow termination point to 50-75% of peak expiratory flow. In essence it is creating intentional auto-PEEP (not allowing flow to return to baseline during exhalation)*
Trigger	Set to avoid auto-triggering; may require pressure trigger
Pressure Support	Use of any pressure support is debated. While it may decrease work of breathing, it can also lead to higher transpulmonary pressures (including ↑ risk of overdistension which would offset any gains in V/Q matching)

Modes

APRV Recruitment (Non-Rescue) Initial Settings

P$_{high}$ (high pressure level)	15-30 cmH$_2$O The lower the patient's P/F ratio (or higher the OI), the higher the initial setting needed
T$_{high}$ (time spent at high pressure level)	~4-6 sec (longer than with rescue with the goal of maximizing CPAP and therefore recruitment)
P$_{low}$ (low pressure level)	0 cmH$_2$O Allows for maximum ΔP for unimpeded expiratory flow. Setting above zero may add expiratory resistance, inhibiting CO$_2$ removal (the lungs are kept open using T$_{low}$, not P$_{low}$)
T$_{low}$ (time spent at low pressure level)	The actual value is less important than using ventilator graphics Typically ~0.2-0.6 seconds (75% of PEF) *Use flow scalar or loop to set expiratory flow termination point to 50-75% of peak expiratory flow. In essence it is creating intentional auto-PEEP (not allowing flow to return to baseline during exhalation)*
Trigger	Set to avoid auto-triggering; may require pressure trigger
Pressure Support	Use of any pressure support is debated (and often not recommended). While it may decrease work of breathing, it can also lead to higher transpulmonary pressures (including ↑ risk of overdistension which would offset any gains in V/Q matching)

Modes

Improving Oxygenation on APRV (Goal: ↑ PaO₂)

P high (high pressure level)	**Increase** in 2-5 cmH₂O increments (up to 30, maybe 40 with low compliance). Monitor hemodynamic status.
T high (time spent at high pressure level)	**Increase** by 0.5-2 sec, along with P high increases (may go up to 10-15 seconds)
T low (time spent at low pressure level)	**Decrease** T low in 0.1 sec increments towards expiratory flow termination of 75% of PEF (increases end expiratory lung volume). Caution: May decrease V$_T$, which will ↑ CO₂
FIO₂	Keep FIO₂ as low as clinically indicated
Recruitment	Consider recruitment maneuvers if necessary (e.g. P high 40-50 cmH₂O and T high 30-60 sec)

Improving Ventilation on APRV (Goal: ↓ $PaCO_2$)

Phigh (high pressure level)	**Increase** in 2-5 cmH₂O increments (up to 30, maybe 40 with low compliance). Increases ΔP, increasing expiratory flow and CO_2 elimination. Monitor tidal volume and hemodynamic status.
Thigh (time spent at high pressure level)	**Preferred Method:** **Increase** Thigh in 0.5-1 increments, along with Phigh increases (may go up to 10-15 seconds). Monitor VT/hemo status. It increases minute ventilation by increasing ΔP, while preserving FRC (the Thigh, in part, does this) **Less Preferred Method (do preferred first!):** **Decrease** Thigh in 0.5-0.1 increments simultaneously with increasing Phigh. This increases minute ventilation by allowing for more releases, but may decrease mPAW (affecting oxygenation).
Tlow (time spent at low pressure level)	**TCAV (rescue): maintain at 75% PEF** **Increase** Tlow in 0.1 increments towards 50% PEF to allow more time for exhalation. This may lead to airway closure/derecruitment (oxygenation status should be acceptable)

Improving Ventilation on APRV (Goal: ↑ $PaCO_2$)

Phigh (high pressure level)	**Decrease** in 2-5 cmH₂O increments if oxygenation status is acceptable. This decreases ΔP, decreasing expiratory flow and CO_2 elimination.
Thigh (time spent at high pressure level)	**Increase** slowly in increments of 0.5-2 seconds. This reduces number of releases.

Weaning APRV

1. **Wean FiO₂ first.** Target is < 50%. Maintain P$_{High}$ for a period of time (24-hrs is recommended) to optimize recruitment
2. **"Drop and Stretch"**
   Do these simultaneously:

DROP P$_{high}$ (high pressure level) **AND**	**Decrease** in 2-5 cmH$_2$O increments ONLY after FiO$_2$ < 50% and oxygenation status stable for 2 hours. Continue until 16-20 cmH$_2$O (maintaining desired PaCO$_2$) This all results in lower mPAW
STRETCH T$_{high}$ (time spent at high pressure level)	**Increase** T$_{high}$ in 0.5 sec increments, up to 15 seconds. This decreases the number of releases and allows for a greater time for spontaneous ventilation during T$_{high}$. At 15 seconds, the release rate is only 4/min - minimal.

3. Reach CPAP

Note that some clinicians transition to a conventional mode of ventilation, such as PSV at this time.

- The goal is to progress towards pure CPAP, by decreasing P$_{high}$ and increasing T$_{high}$ (Drop and Stretch).
- The patient's spontaneous rate should be increasing to compensate
- When P$_{high}$ is around 16 with T$_{high}$ of 12-15 seconds, switch to CPAP
- Titrate CPAP down
- Consider extubation when CPAP 5-10 cmH$_2$O

Volume-Assured Pressure Support (VAPS)	
Summary	Breaths start out as pressure supported (pressure added to each spontaneous breath), but as inspiratory flow begins to decrease, the ventilator checks the delivered volume against a target V_T that the clinician has set. If the volume is adequate, the ventilator cycles into exhalation. If the volume is too low, the ventilator maintains flow until that set volume has been delivered. May be used with A/C, SIMV, or CPAP

	Classified By:		
Breath Type	**Trigger**	**Limit**	**Cycle**
V_T met spontaneously	Patient (flow or pressure)	Vent (pressure)	Patient (flow)
V_T analyzed as not being met spontaneously		Vent (volume)	Vent (volume)

Indications
- Spontaneously breathing patients who require minimum V_T
- Patients who are dyssynchronous with the ventilator
- Used as a back-up for pressure support ventilation (to ensure a minimum V_T for each breath)

VAPS

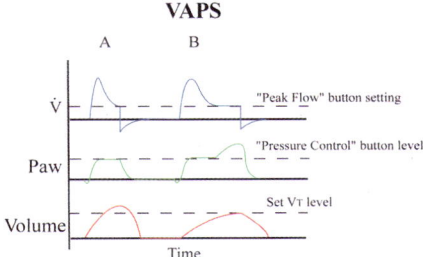

A: Depicts a PS-like breath that has been terminated at the set peak flow after the minimum V_T has been achieved

B: Depicts a transition from a PS-like breath to a volume assured (controlled) breath. Transition occurs when flow has decelerated to the set "Peak Flow" and the set V_T has not been delivered. The I-time is extended until the set V_T is delivered.

How it works:
- When a VAPS breath is delivered, the breath is delivered using whatever pressure level is set ("Pressure Control" button on the front panel).
- If the set minimum V_T is achieved by the time the flow ↓ to the set flow-cycle value ("Peak Flow" button on the front panel), the ventilator cycles into exhalation. In this case, the breath acts as a normal PS breath. The V_T could be exceeded.
- If the set V_T is not achieved, the flow is maintained as a constant flow pattern at the set "peak flow" value until the set V_T is achieved. The breath then acts as a volume-cycled breath.
- If the breath becomes a volume-cycled breath, the resulting pressure will be higher than the set pressure support level

Note: Determining the correct pressure level is complex with no evidence to support any one level over another

Clinical Notes
- Volume is guaranteed for each breath
- Potentially decreased work of breathing
- Choosing the appropriate pressure and flow settings are critical for successful and safe operation.
  Examples:
  - If the "peak flow" (flow-cycle value) is set too high, all the breaths will switch from pressure to volume-cycled, which will defeat the purpose of using the mode
  - If the "peak flow" is set too low, the inspiratory time could be too long to achieve the desired set V_T and I:E
  - If the pressure is set too high, the volume back-up will never be needed
  - If the pressure is set too low and/or the V_T is set too low, the patient could become distressed and/or under-ventilated
- A sudden increase in spontaneous rate and demand may result in a decrease in ventilatory support

Pressure-Regulated Volume Control
(PRVC)

Summary	This is a variable pressure mode with a set target tidal volume. The ventilator titrates the pressure, breath-by-breath, to attempt to reach the set VT. A high pressure alarm is set which then acts as a limit (prevents excessive pressures when set correctly)

	Classified By:		
Breath Type	**Trigger**	**Limit**	**Cycle**
Assisted	Patient (flow or pressure)	Vent (pressure or volume)	Vent (time = TI)
Controlled	Vent (time = rate)	Vent (pressure or volume)	Vent (time = TI)

How it Works
- For the first breath, the ventilator gives a volume breath with a pause (plateau)
- The second breath will be a pressure breath at that plateau pressure from the previous breath
- The ventilator will then titrate the inspiratory pressure by no more than 3 cmH$_2$O from one breath to the next in order to try to meet the target VT
- As a safety, the maximum available pressure level is 5 cmH$_2$O below the preset upper pressure alarm (alarm will sound at this point and the breath will switch into exhalation, meaning the set VT will not be fully delivered - the ventilator will only deliver the amount of volume that it can before hitting that upper limit)
- The minimum inspiratory pressure limit is the baseline setting (PEEP)
- PRVC can be combined with SIMV so that mandatory breaths are PRVC, spontaneous breaths are pressure supported

Modes

PRVC

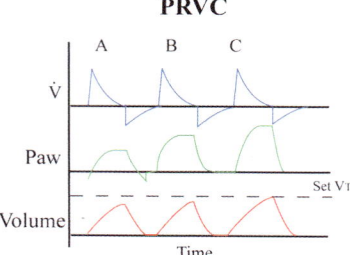

As the breaths advance from A to C, the pressure is automatically increased to achieve the set V_T.

Indications:
Indications are similar to Pressure A/C

Clinical Notes
- Tidal volume and minute ventilation are guaranteed (unless breaths are pressure-limiting due to high PIPs - or high pressure alarm set too low)
- Allows patient control of RR and $\dot{V}_E$
- Variable $\dot{V}_I$ (decelerating) to meet patient demand and potentially improve gas distribution
- The high pressure alarm also serves as a high pressure limit, making it critical that this is set correctly
- Patients who assist the ventilator by taking larger breaths will cause the inspiratory pressure to drop (as the ventilator drops it in increments of 3s to try to get to goal V_T). If the patient then tires, the ventilator could be delivering as low as the PEEP level at a time when the patient most needs the support. A PIP dropping to PEEP level is a warning of this risk.
- Other clinical causes may cause pressure-limiting of breaths (meaning the target tidal volume is not met) include excessive coughing, fighting/breathing against the vent, hiccups, low C or high Raw. Consider treating underlying causes or consider a different mode.

Adaptive Pressure Ventilation
(APV)

Summary	See PRVC for details. The following differences exist: pressure is titrated in 1 cmH$_2$O increments (versus 3 in PRVC); maximum pressure is 10 cmH$_2$O below high Pressure alarm (versus 5), and low pressure is 5 cm H$_2$O above set PEEP (versus none).

	Classified By:		
Breath Type	**Trigger**	**Limit**	**Cycle**
Assisted	Patient (flow or pressure)	Vent (pressure or volume)	Vent (time = TI)
Controlled	Vent (time = rate)	Vent (pressure or volume)	Vent (time = TI)

Operation
- The ventilator continuously calculates system and patient Compliance, and volume delivery
- If the exhaled V$_T$ is less or more than the set V$_T$, the inspiratory pressure level is regulated until the preset volumes are delivered. Pressure changes are made in 1 cmH$_2$O increments
- Maximum available inspiratory pressure level is 10 cmH$_2$O below the set upper pressure limit
- The amount of pressure cannot be set lower than 5 cmH$_2$O above the baseline pressure (PEEP)
- The patient will receive a minimum number of time-triggered mandatory breaths per minute (Set back-up rate)

Clinical Notes
See PRVC for relevant clinical notes

Proportional Assist Ventilation
Proportional Pressure Support
(PAV, PPS)

Summary	Mode delivers flow, volume, and pressure based upon the patient's needs (as determined by patient effort), at a percentage set by the clinician. The goal is to standardize the patient's WOB.

	Classified By:		
Breath Type	Trigger	Limit	Cycle
Assisted	Patient (flow or pressure)	Vent (pressure)	Vent (flow)

Operation
- The ventilator continuously calculates system and patient compliance, and volume delivery
- If the exhaled V_T is less or more than the set V_T, the inspiratory pressure level is regulated until the preset volumes are delivered. Pressure changes are made in 1 cmH_2O increments
- Maximum available inspiratory pressure level is 10 cmH_2O below the set upper pressure limit
- The amount of pressure cannot be set lower than 5 cmH_2O above the baseline pressure (PEEP)
- The patient will receive a minimum number of time-triggered mandatory breaths per minute (Set back-up rate)

Clinical Notes
May be used with any Volume mode (V-A/C, V-SIMV, and V-MMV), but changes <u>volume</u> to <u>pressure</u> with volume target
- The expiratory valve is floating, which allows the patient to cough or breathe during the inspiratory time of the mandatory breath while maintaining the achieved inspiratory pressure without a significant undershoot or overshoot

Modes

PAV

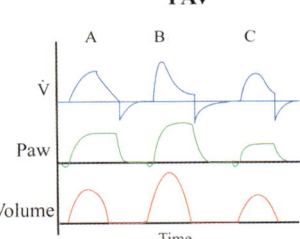

The effort and pressure are increased in Breath B compared to Breath A. The effort and pressure are decreased in Breath C.

Indications:
- High work of breathing with worsening lung characteristics
- Asynchronous patients who are stable with an inspiratory effort
- Ventilator-dependent patients with COPD

Advantages:
- The patient controls the ventilatory variables ($\dot{V}_I$, PIP, T_I, T_E, V_T)
- Trends the changes of ventilatory effort over time
- When used with CPAP, inspiratory muscle work is near that of a normal subject and may decrease or prevent muscle atrophy
- Lowers airway pressures

Disadvantages and Risks:
- Patient must have adequate spontaneous respiratory drive
- Variable V_T and/or PIP
- Excessive assist ("Runaway") by the ventilator may occur (High V_T and pressure alarms must be set appropriately)
- Air leak could cause excessive assist or automatic cycling
- Trigger effort may increase with auto-PEEP
- Backup mode required in case of apnea
- Correct determination of compliance and resistance is essential, yet difficult. Both under and over estimates of C and Raw (or changes in C and Raw, as with repositioning) may significantly impair proper patient-ventilator interaction

SmartCare Pressure Support

Summary	A closed system weaning mode that automatically titrates pressure support levels based on tidal volume, spontaneous rate, and end-tidal CO_2

How It Works:
- There are 3 sets of values based on actual body weight
- Each body weight range (15-35 kg, 26-55 kg, and over 55 kg) has different criteria for acceptable tidal volume and frequency
- Based on the patient's initial frequency, tidal volume and $ETCO_2$, Smartcare assigns the patient's ventilation to one of eight categories: normal ventilation, insufficient ventilation, hypoventilation, central hypoventilation, tachypnea, severe tachypnea, hyperventilation, or unexplained hyperventilation.
- The clinician also may select "COPD" or "Neurological Disorder" to allow different acceptable parameters (eg., higher $ETCO_2$)
- Ventilation other than normal will increase or decrease PS by 2-4 cmH$_2$O (based upon which parameter is out-of-range)
- Smartcare assesses the patient's RR, V$_T$ and $ETCO_2$ every 10 seconds and analyzes ventilation every two minutes if there was no PS change or every 5 minutes if there was a PS change
- When the target pressure is obtained, a spontaneous breathing test is performed and if predetermined weight-based values are met a message "SC-Consider Separation" is displayed suggesting to the clinician that liberation may be possible

Indications:
- Spontaneously breathing patients weighing 15-200 kg
- Patients who meet criteria for weaning

Advantages:
- Ability to have patient frequently assessed mechanically
- Documented improved weaning times

Disadvantages and Risks:
- Clinician must still use bedside assessment and judgment
- $ETCO_2$ results will be inaccurate if any V/Q mismatch present

Volume Support
(VS)

Summary	A spontaneous breathing mode with a variable amount of pressure support (determined by a target/set tidal volume)

	Classified By:		
Breath Type	**Trigger**	**Limit**	**Cycle**
Supported	Patient (flow or pressure)	Patient (pressure or volume)	Patient (flow or time)

Operation

- The ventilator gives a test breath with an inspiratory pressure of 10 cmH$_2$O above PEEP
- The volume delivered is measured, then system compliance is calculated
- For each subsequent breath, the ventilator calculates compliance of the previous breath and adjusts the inspiratory pressure level (pressure support) to achieve the set V$_T$ on the next breath
- The maximum change is 3 cmH$_2$O from one breath to the next
- Maximum available inspiratory pressure level is 5 cmH$_2$O below the preset upper pressure limit (alarm will sound at this point and the breath will switch into exhalation)
- The minimum pressure limit is the baseline setting (PEEP)
- If apnea occurs, back up pressure support is activated and an alarm sounds
- If Automode is on and patient becomes apneic, the mode will automatically switch to PRVC (See Automode)

Modes

VS

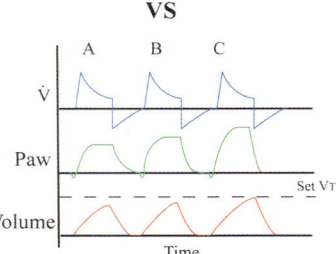

In this example, as the breaths advance from A to C, the pressure is automatically increased to achieve the set V_T. All breaths are patient-triggered breaths.

Indications:
- Spontaneous breathing patients who require minimum V_T
- Patients who have inspiratory efforts who need added support
- Patients who are asynchronous with the ventilator
- Used for patients who are ready to wean

Advantages:
- Guaranteed V_T and $\dot{V}_E$
- Pressure supported breaths using the lowest required pressure
- Decreases the patient's spontaneous RR and WOB
- Allows patient control of inspiratory and expiratory Times (and I:E ratio)
- Variable $\dot{V}_I$ to meet the patient's demand

Disadvantages and Risks:
- Spontaneous ventilation required
- Auto-PEEP may affect operation
- Patients who assist the ventilator by taking larger V_T will cause the inspiratory pressure to drop (as the ventilator drops it in increments of 3s to try to get to goal V_T). If the patient then tires, the ventilator could be delivering as low as the PEEP level at a time when the patient most needs the support. A PIP dropping to PEEP level is a warning of this likelihood.

Modes

Adaptive Support Ventilation
(ASV, AVtS)

Summary	A closed-system, dual control mode that uses pressure ventilation (both pressure control and pressure support) to maintain a minimum minute ventilation using the least required settings for minimal WOB

	Classified By:		
Breath Type	**Trigger**	**Limit**	**Cycle**
Supported	Patient (flow or pressure)	Patient (pressure)	Patient (flow, pressure, or time)
Mandatory	Ventilator (time = rate)	Ventilator (pressure)	Ventilator (time = TI)

Operation
- The patient's ideal body weight (kg) is entered
- The ventilator delivers 100/mL/min/kg
- A guaranteed minute ventilation is set: from 20-200%. This determines the pressure control contribution that will be added if patient doesn't adequately contribute it spontaneously
- Test breaths measure system compliance, resistance, auto-PEEP
- If no spontaneous breaths: a f, VT, and pressure limit deliver for mandatory breaths (I:E ratio and TI are also being optimized)
- As the patient initiates breaths, the ventilator delivers PS at the same pressure level as the mandatory breaths were, while the number of mandatory breaths decreases
- The spontaneous + mandatory breaths are combined to meet the minute ventilation target

Clinical Notes
- In theory, the ventilator adapts to the patient, allowing for automatic/continuous wean (closed-loop)
- Sudden changes in demand (RR) may result in an inadequate immediate response by the ventilator

Continuous Positive Airway Pressure (CPAP)	
Summary	Spontaneous mode with a constant pressure delivered during both inspiration and expiration.

	Classified By:		
Breath Type	**Trigger**	**Limit**	**Cycle**
Spontaneous	Patient (flow or pressure)	Patient (pressure)	Patient (pressure or flow)

Indications
- Spontaneously breathing patients, usually for SBTs

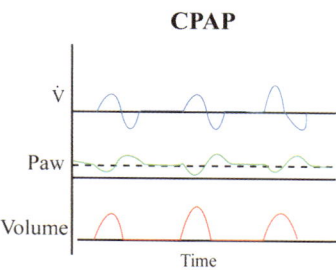

CPAP

Clinical Notes
- No ventilatory support is provided (an independent drive to breathe is required with adequate tidal volume and rate)
- Oxygenation may improve if hypoxemia is due to low lung volumes/atelectasis
- Excessive CPAP level increases risk of air trapping and increases expiratory work of breathing
- CPAP does not compensate for resistance of the artificial airway. Many clinicians prefer pressure support, even if PS is set at minimal levels (PSV 10/5, for example), for this reason.

Automatic Tube Compensation
(ATC)

Summary	This is technically an adjunct, not a mode. The goal of ATC is to overcome the work of breathing caused by an artificial airway. A variable pressure support is provided (more during inspiration than expiration), which is proportional to the inspiratory flow and the internal diameter of the ET tube (as entered into the ventilator).

Operation
- Endotracheal tube size is entered into vent as well as a percentage of compensation desired (1%-100%). The vent then monitors inspiratory flow.
- The airway pressure (PS) is increased during inspiration and decreased during expiration to overcome the resistance (the expiratory portion can be disabled)
- This assisting pressure occurs during exhalation of any ventilator breaths and during both phases of spontaneous breaths
- The delivered pressure ranges from 0 cmH$_2$O up to 5 cmH$_2$O below the set upper pressure limit

Clinical Notes
- The goal of ATC is to overcome the resistance of the artificial airway. This is independent of supporting patient's needs.
- Compensation may be less than expected with any kinks or bends in the airway, or with secretions
- In patients with obstructive lung diseases, small airways may be kept open by PEEP ET tube resistance. Consider setting ATC to be inactive during the expiratory phase.
- Adding ATC to another mode may result in over assist, in which case, the primary support level may need to be reduced. This needs to be particularly noted during weaning attempts (SBT) using Pressure Support as the patient is potentially receiving more PS than what is "dialed in" to the ventilator (ATC adds variable PS to the already set PS)

Automode

Summary	Automode switches between controlled modes (PRVC, Pressure A/C, Volume A/C) and spontaneous modes (PS, VS). When the patient triggers a breath, they breathe on the spontaneous/supported mode; when the patient fails to trigger (apnea, etc.), they breathe on the mandatory side.

Indications
- Patients with a spontaneous drive to breathe that have met criteria for weaning readiness

Operation
- While in the controlled mode: if the patient consecutively triggers the vent twice, the ventilator will transition to support mode.
- While in the spontaneous/supported mode: If the patient fails to trigger a breath over a period of time (varies, but is generally around 12-seconds in adults), the ventilator will transition to the controlled mode.

Controlled Mode	Pt triggers 2x in a row ⇄ apneic period	Spontaneous (Support) Mode
Volume Control	⇄	Volume Support
Pressure Control	⇄	Pressure Support
PRVC	⇄	Volume Support

Clinical Notes
- Trigger must be set carefully as it determines support (if patient can't trigger, a controlled mode will be inappropriately maintained. If the vent auto-triggers, this may be dangerously interpreted as spontaneous breaths)
- If switching to volume support, the ventilator determines inspiratory pressure using a formula: Set P = ([PIP-PEEP] x 0.5 + PEEP)
- Information on each mode can be found in that mode's topic

Neurally Adjusted Ventilatory Assist
(NAVA, NIV-NAVA)

Summary	This <u>noninvasive or invasive</u> mode incorporates neural triggering (through a sensor on a specialized nasogastric catheter positioned in the esophagus near the diaphragm) with spontaneous breaths that are pressure supported proportionally to the strength of the electrical signal from the diaphragm.

	Classified By:		
Breath Type	**Trigger**	**Limit**	**Cycle**
Spontaneous (NAVA)	Patient (neural, pressure, or flow)	Patient (neural)	Patient (neural)
Spontaneous (PS)	Patient (pressure or flow)	Patient (pressure)	Patient (flow, pressure, or time)
Mandatory	Ventilator (time = rate)	Ventilator (pressure)	Ventilator (time = TI)
Assisted	Assisted breaths will return pt to NAVA		

How It Works:
- A specialized nasogastric (NG) tube with an array of electrodes (Edi catheter) is positioned in the esophagus to optimally detect the electrical activity of the diaphragm
- An Edi positioning screen utilizes a 4-channel retrocardiac ECG pattern to assist the clinician on the **proper placement** of the Edi catheter. Correct NG catheter position is demonstrated by the largest p-waves and by the QRS complexes being present in the upper leads and subsequently progressing to minimal or absent p-waves. QRS complexes remain present in the lower leads.
- The Edi signal is superimposed on the retrocardiac ECG as a blue color and should be on the second and third lead but may periodically fluctuate to the upper and lower leads without loss of signal integrity. A trigger level is set. Once the threshold is reached (Edi min + Trigger level), **a breath is initiated.**
- **The ventilator assists the spontaneous breath** of the patient by delivering pressure directly and linearly proportional to the Edi or neural respiratory drive. Inspiration (pressure delivery) is proportionally maintained until the electrical activity decreases by 30% and the breath is then terminated. This allows the patient to determine inspiratory pressure (or volume), inspiratory and expiratory time, and respiratory rate for each breath.
- The clinician sets a **backup pressure support level** with trigger and cycle off criteria so the patient can flow-trigger the ventilator should the Edi catheter become displaced. Neural respiratory rate and timing can differ from the pneumatic rate and time. This may be caused by well known pneumatic/flow trigger challenges including delayed, false, or missed triggering.
- **In case of apnea** (absent Edi signal and pneumatic triggers that last longer than an adjustable apnea time limit), the ventilator will switch to standard pressure control ventilation (NAVA backup). This adjustable apnea time acts as a minimum rate and can be adjusted from as little as 2 seconds (min. rate 30 breaths/min) to 30 seconds (min. rate 2 breaths /min). **Once the patient starts breathing spontaneously, the ventilator will switch back to a NAVA mode.**

Indications:
- Mode is used in neonatal-to-adult populations
- Edi monitoring alone may be done on any patient in any mode of ventilation. This can be used as another respiratory vital sign and gives information about neural respiratory drive, work of breathing, response to sedation, and synchrony in non-NAVA modes.
- Spontaneously breathing patients can be ventilated on NAVA even when having prolonged periods of apnea. Patients should not be paralyzed, overly sedated, or over-ventilated.
- Patients who are dyssynchronous on conventional modes of ventilation

Proposed Advantages:
- Reduces work of breathing—less missed patient trigger efforts. Intrinsic PEEP will not affect triggering in NAVA
- Improves synchrony—the patient's neural trigger controls onset, breath size (pressure and volume) and cycling off of each breath. Ventilator synchrony with the patient is an important part of unloading the work of the diaphragm during both inspiration and expiration.
- May reduce need for sedation/paralysis—by allowing the patient to control their own breathing pattern, less sedation may be required
- May improve ventilation—compared to standard methods, by allowing neural triggering, cycling and neurally-adjusted ventilator assistance (e.g., patients with severe airflow impairment)
- May reduce overall peak inspiratory pressures being delivered (patients get the pressure they need for that breath)

Disadvantages and Risks:
- Correct placement of the NG catheter is important but easily maintained and monitored. Any significant displacement will interfere with the mode (a backup system as outlined above is in place) and an alarm alerts the provider to reassess catheter position.
- Cannot be used if the respiratory center, phrenic nerve and neuromuscular junction are not intact or are chemically depressed
- The respiratory drive (Edi signal) may not be present if patient is over-ventilated. This may be a result of too high NAVA level or too much backup support.

Edi Catheter (same catheter for both invasive and noninvasive)

- Edi signal is in microvolts (μv)
- The phrenic nerve activates the diaphragm electrically. Edi is a representation of this signal.
- There is generally more variability in phases and baseline in infant Edi signals as compared to adult Edi signals
- Increased Edi amplitude (phasic Edi) indicates greater inspiratory effort
- Approved by U.S. FDA as a functioning NG/OG tube

Edi amplitude increases	Edi amplitude decreases
worsening resp. status ↓ ventilator assist ↓ sedation ↑ deadspace ↑ ventilatory demand (e.g., crying, moving, etc.)	improving resp. status ↑ ventilator assist ↑ sedation ↓ deadspace

Breath Start ➔ (Trigger)	During Breath ➔	Breath End (Cycle)
Edi Trigger Level (which is set) is reached which initiates ...	... an assist <u>in proportion to</u> the Edi signal. This is provided until...	... the Edi signal has fallen to 70% of its peak value, at which time passive exhalation is allowed
Edi Trigger Level	**Pressure delivered (PIP) =** NAVA level x (Edi signal - Edi min) + PEEP	

Modes

Insertion and Positioning of the Edi Catheter

Height	Weight	Edi Catheter Size	Inter-Electrode Distance (IED)
45-35 cm	--	8 FR 100 cm	8mm
< 55 cm	1.0 - 2.0 kg	6 FR 50 cm	6 mm
< 55 cm	0.5 - 1.5 kg	6 FR 49 cm	6 mm

1. Take NEX Measurement. This is the distance from the bridge of the nose to the earlobe to the xiphoid process.

2. Calculate insertion distance (NEX is measurement from #1)

	Nasal (in Y cm)	Oral (in Y cm)
8 FR 100 cm	NEX cm x 0.9 + 8	NEX cm x 0.8 + 8
6 FR 50 cm	NEX cm x 0.9 + 3.5	NEX cm x 0.8 + 3.5
6 FR 49 cm	NEX cm x 0.9 + 2.5	NEX cm x 0.8 + 2.5

3. D p Edi catheter into water - DO NOT USE LUBRICANT
   Insert the catheter to the Y distance from #2

4. Connect catheter to cable

5. Verify positioning of the catheter
   ECG: P, QRS present in top leads
   P waves decrease and disappear; QRS decreases
   If 2nd and 3rd leads are highlighted in blue: secure
   If top leads are highlighted in blue: withdraw to the inter-electrode distance (IED)
   If bottom leads are constantly highlighted in blue: insert further

Modes

Typical Invasive NAVA Initial Settings (specific to this mode)

NAVA level	0-4 cmH$_2$O/µV
	1. Start at a NAVA level of 2 cmH$_2$O/ µV and evaluate the WOB
	2. If ↑ WOB (and associated high Edi peaks) increase the NAVA level in 0.5 cmH2O/ µV increments until the patient is comfortable and the Edi peaks are 5-15 µV. Maintain.
	3. If the patient is comfortable and the Edi peaks are < 5 µV, decrease the NAVA level in 0.5 cmH$_2$O/ µV increments until the Edi peak mostly are > 5 µV or the patient begins to work harder.
Trigger Edi	Default = 0.5 µV (range = 0-2 µV)
NAVA PS	Ensure adequate PS: Set the PS at the same level as PC in the backup settings
Back-Up	***Ensure Adequate Back-Up:*** **Mode**: Pressure Control **Inspiratory Pressure**: set high enough to move the chest (typically 15-25 cmH$_2$O)
Peak Pressure Limit	Set high enough to allow recruiting breaths (35-40 cmH$_2$O); ↑ if upper limit is alarming
Apnea Time	Set short enough that the patient gets a rescue (backup) breath before any clinical decompensation is noted. This represents minimum ventilator rate.

Weaning

- Once WOB is minimal, Edi peaks < 15 µV, and blood gas is acceptable (pH > 7.25, PCO$_2$ < 60, O$_2$% < 30), decrease NAVA level in 0.5 cmH$_2$O/ µV increments until the Edi peaks rise, or the patient WOB increases. Attempt 2-3 times/day or as tolerated.
- When at NAVA level of 1 cmH$_2$O/ µV, consider extubation to NIV NAVA, increasing the NAVA level back to 2 cmH$_2$O/ µV and titrating to the appropriate level as described above.
- Patients with chronic lung disease may require less frequent and smaller incremental changes in NAVA level.

Invasive NAVA: How Modes are Automatically Selected[1]

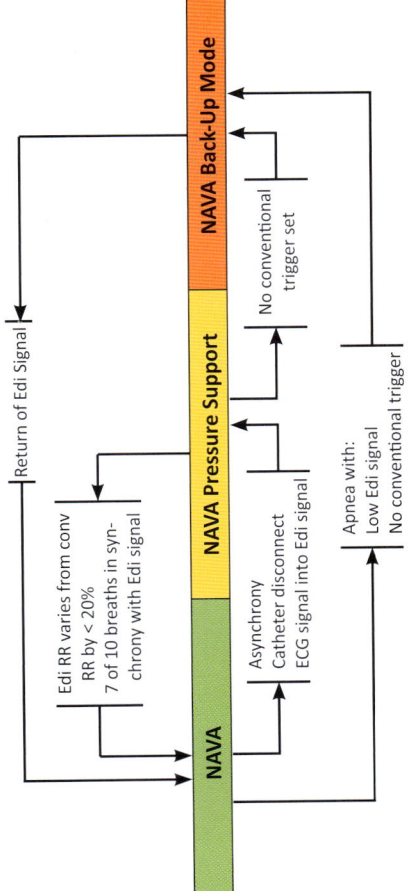

[1]Adapted from Maquet, Inc.: NAVA and NIV NAVA Neonatal Pocket Guide

Noninvasive NAVA Initial Settings (specific to this mode)

NAVA level	0-4 cmH$_2$O/ μV. Default = 2 Start with NAVA level at 2 and adjust as described for invasive NAVA
Trigger Edi	Default = 0.5 μV (range = 0-2 μV)
Back-Up	***Ensure Adequate Back-Up:*** **Mode**: Pressure Control **Inspiratory Pressure**: set high enough to move the chest (typically 20-25 cmH$_2$O) **Rate**: set at 40-60 breaths/min **Inspiratory Time**: 0.35-0.4 second
Peak Pressure Limit	Set high enough to allow recruiting breaths (35-40 cmH$_2$O); ↑ if upper limit is alarming
Apnea Time	Set short enough that the patient gets a rescue (backup) breath before any clinical decompensation is noted.

Weaning
- Use same approach as with Invasive NAVA
- When NAVA level is 1 cmH$_2$O/uV, consider transition to CPAP

NAVA Troubleshooting

Issue	Possible Problem(s)	Possible Correction(s)
No or low Edi signal	Over-ventilation Over-sedation Central apnea	Verify muscle relaxants worn off Verify patient's sedation level Verify patient is not hyperventilated Review blood gas/EtCO$_2$
Stays in NAVA (Backup) mode (no neural or pneumatic trigger)	Over-ventilation Over-sedation Central apnea	Decrease ventilation and monitor Decrease sedation and monitor Consider changing ventilator mode
Stays in NAVA (PS) mode	Most commonly from a large air leak	Make the flow trigger less sensitive Reintubate with a larger ET tube Change to NIV NAVA used invasively
Alarm: Pneumatic-Edi out of synch	**Specific cases of asynchrony:** • Edi RR differs from pneumatic RR with > 25% for at least 5 seconds (calculated RR based on last 20 seconds) • Edi TI/TTOT > 0.5 seconds (calculated over last 20 seconds) • Edi catheter disconnected • ECG leakage through Edi signal	Check Edi signal Ensure proper catheter position Troubleshoot in this order: 1. ↓ pneumatic trigger setting 2. Adjust (↑ or ↓) the Edi trigger in increments of 0.1 uV 3. Adjust inspiratory cycle off setting

Modes

Issue	Possible Problem(s)	Possible Correction(s)
Respiratory acidosis in infants with apnea of prematurity who are experiencing multiple apneic episodes per minute	• Insufficient backup support when patient is in the NAVA (backup) mode • Apnea time is too long	Increase set backup rate and/or PC above PEEP Shorten apnea time
Edi Monitoring not active message	NAVA mode is activated without the Edi module being connected	Connect and perform the Edi Module test
Edi Module disconnected message *Edi Module error* message	Edi module is not properly installed	Reinsert module and perform the Edi Module test
Check Edi catheter position message	Edi catheter not in appropriate position	Check Edi catheter positioning screen and reposition Edi catheter as needed
Peak Inspiratory Pressure alarm	Peak pressure limit set too low	Assess patient Increase peak pressure limit
Edi min is consistently higher than 3.0	This may be an indication that additional PEEP is needed	Consider increasing PEEP

Extracorporeal Membrane Oxygenation
(ECMO, ECCO$_2$R))

Summary	Blood is circulated out of the body (through cannulization), where it is run through artificial membranes (diffusion, hollow-fiber), allowing for molecular oxygen and carbon dioxide diffusion. The blood then re-enters the body through another cannula.
Goal	Allow time for the intrinsic recovery of the lungs and/or heart, or provide the means to medically maintain the patient until organ transplantation is possible. The amount of rest the systems receive is dependent in part on the type of support being provided (see next page).
Techniques	• Extracorporeal Membrane Oxygenation (ECMO) • Extracorporeal Carbon Dioxide Removal (ECCO$_2$R)

Types of Support

Venoarterial (VA) *provides heart and lung support*:

Deoxygenated Blood	actively pumped through oxygenator	Oxygenated Blood
Venous Blood		**Arterial Blood Supply**
Right Atrium	O_2 diffuses in CO_2 diffuses out	Ascending aorta (Central ECMO)
Internal Jugular Vein		Internal Carotid Artery

- Decreases cardiac work
- Decreases cardiac oxygen consumption
- Proportion of blood flow can continue through lungs

Venovenous (VV) *provides lung support*:

Deoxygenated Blood	actively pumped through oxygenator	Oxygenated Blood
Venous Blood		**Venous Blood Supply**
Single Dual-Lumen Cannula in the Internal Jugular Vein		Single Dual-Lumen Cannula in the Internal Jugular Vein
Blood enters the cannula through the lower port (usually in Inferior Vena Cava)	O_2 diffuses in CO_2 diffuses out	Blood exits the cannula through the proximal port (usually in the right atrium)

- Does not support circulation
- May recirculate previously oxygenated blood (depends on cannula placement)
- $ECCO_2R$ allows for oxygenation by lungs, CO_2 removal by ECMO
- Femoral access is not indicated in children < 10 kg

Relative Contraindications
- Evidence of ischemic neurological damage
- Structural (congenital) cardiac disease
- Severe hypoxemia (prolonged)
- Mechanical ventilation (prolonged > 7 days)

Absolute Contraindications
- Weight < 2 kg and/or age < 35 wks gestational
- Severe asphyxia or ischemia
- Poor underlying prognosis (trisomy 13, trisomy 18, etc.)
- Anticoagulation contraindications (numerous)

Ventilator Management

Patient / Goal	Typical Settings
Cardiac patients Goal: maintain lung function near normal	Pressure Assist/Control PIP ~ 25 cmH$_2$O (VT 5-7 mL/kg IBW) PEEP 5 cmH$_2$O f: 10-12 breaths/min
Respiratory patients Goal: allow lungs to rest while preventing atelectasis.	Pressure Assist/Control PIP ~20-25 cmH$_2$O (VT 4-6 mL/kg IBW) PEEP 4-10 cmH$_2$O f: 4-10 breaths/min

- For <u>vent rest</u>: once vent support is set, generally ABGs are managed on the ECMO side (don't fix with the ventilator)
- With VV ECMO SpO$_2$ will be lower (> 85%)
- Wean ventilator FIO$_2$ once stabilized on ECMO
- "Whited out" CXR is expected for first 24-hours of support

ECMO Weaning/discontinuation
- Weaning is the gradual reduction of ECMO *blood flow* and *sweep gas rates* over a period of hours-to-days with simultaneous increase in ventilatory support (as ECMO flow decreases, ventilator settings, including FIO$_2$, will need to increase as more blood is circulating naturally).
- When flow rates reach 10-30 mL/kg/min, the patient may be isolated from the ECMO circuit
- Alternatively, a trial separation from ECMO support may be performed (with appropriate ventilator support)

Modes

High-Frequency Oscillatory Ventilation
(HFOV)

Summary	Often referred to as "the oscillator" or "oscillation"
	A Mean Airway Pressure (mPAW) is set to keep the airways/alveoli open (like CPAP does), and then very small breaths (which are less than deadspace) are delivered at very high rates
	Inspiration and exhalation are both active (this is unusual as exhalation is passive in most modes of ventilation)
	Note that there is clinical debate on the use of HFOV in adults, with benefits being primarily around lung protection and recruitment with severe ARDS, while concerns center around the knowledge needed to operate an oscillator

	Classified By*:		
Breath Type	**Trigger**	**Limit**	**Cycle**
Mandatory	Ventilator (time)	Ventilator (pressure)	Ventilator (time)

*Note that while this technically classifies a breath, HFOV does not utilize conventional breaths for the majority of the alveoli. These small breaths theoretically use passive gas diffusion, pendelluft, asymmetric velocity profiles, turbulence, and other mechanisms of gas flow at very high rates to distribute and exchange gases.

Definitions

mPAW	Mean Airway Pressure, which directly affects Oxygenation. The maximum possible is 55-60 cmH$_2$O
Bias Flow	Flow of gases through circuit which maintains set mean airway pressure. Increasing bias flow will enable an increase in mPAW
Power	Controls electrical current level applied to motor. This setting on the oscillator alters the ΔP which effects CO$_2$ elimination
Amplitude (delta-P)	**Primary determinant of CO$_2$ elimination** HFOV ventilation = $f \times V_T^2$ Conventional ventilation = $f \times V_T$ Changes in V_t affect CO$_2$ more drastically than changes in f
Hertz Hz (Frequency)	**Secondary determinant of CO$_2$ elimination** Number of times the piston moves fully forward and fully backward (1 inhalation + 1 exhalation) Hertz x 60 = Cycles/minute Hertz is inversely proportional to volume (the higher the Hz, the lower the oscillating volumes)
Inspiratory Time	The amount of time the piston is in the forward motion This is set as a % on oscillator (usually 33%)
Expiratory Time	Backward movement of the piston Unlike most modes of ventilation, exhalation is active
Chest Wiggle Factor (CWF)	An informal manner of assessing volume displacement (amplitude/power)

Modes

HFOV (Oscillator)
Suggested Initial Settings
(non-disease specific, based on *Sensormedics/Vyaire 3100B Device*)

Primary Oxygenation	**MAP**	Direct: ~34 cmH$_2$O From Conventional: 2-4 cmH$_2$O above conventional MAP
	Inspiratory Time	33%
	FIO$_2$	Match from conventional (usually 1.0)
Primary Ventilation	**Power**	*Power is set to target ΔP*
	Delta-P (ΔP) Amplitude	~90 cmH$_2$O
	Hertz (Hz)	4-8 Hz (lower Hz for lower pH) Both depend on lung disease. Use higher for restrictive disorders; lower for obstructive disorders.
Other	**Bias Flow (L/min)**	40 L/min Too low: can't reach MAP Too high: prevents full exhalation (↑ CO$_2$)
Sedation	Heavier sedation, sometimes paralytics are necessary to manage a patient on HFOV	

Some clinicians recommend performing a recruitment maneuver after starting the oscillator

Special Note on Ventilation with HFOV:

Power and ΔP are interconnected. Power is a setting on the oscillator which controls ΔP. ΔP is a measurement, and is thus set primarily by the Power setting.

Some clinicians target a specific power setting, allowing ΔP to change in response to compliance/resistance changes in the patient. Other clinicians target a specific ΔP and thus will regularly alter the power setting to ensure the target ΔP.

↑ Power results in ↑ ΔP (↑ ventilation)
↓ Power results in ↓ ΔP (↓ ventilation)

HFOV: Managing and Monitoring

Primary Methods for Adjusting Oxygenation

#1 Optimize Mean Airway Pressure
Oxygenation on the oscillator is primarily targeted by using mPAW. CXR: Goal is convex diaphragms, minimal atelectasis, normal-sized heart. 8-9 ribs posteriorly above diaphragm is used (but may be misleading)

#2 Titrate FiO₂
The goal is to maintain a safe O₂% whenever possible. Optimizing mPAW has greater benefit in the long-term.

Primary Methods for Adjusting Ventilation

Problem: ↑ PaCO₂ = underventilated	
#1 Power/ΔP	Increase ΔP to increase the amplitude (~ size of the breath)
#2 Frequency[1]	↓ Hertz This is counter-intuitive! Reducing frequency ↑ ventilation
#3 Inspiratory Time	Leave at 33% Some clinicians recommend increasing Inspiratory Time to 50% (no higher) for ~10% increase in Vт

Problem: ↓ PaCO₂ = overventilated	
#1 Power/ΔP	Decrease ΔP but ensure adequate chest wiggle
#2 Frequency[1]	↑ Hertz This is counter-intuitive! Increasing Frequency ↓ ventilation

[1] Hertz is rarely changed when it is acceptable for patient size and lung disease.

Modes

Clinical Notes
- An initial CXR should be obtained within 1-2 hours to determine over- and under-expansion based upon heart size, diaphragms, and atelectasis.
- Suctioning (discouraged for first 24-hours unless clinically indicated):
  - diminished chest wall wiggle
  - increasing CO_2
  - decreasing PO_2
  - visible or audible secretions
- Some clinicians stop the piston (start/stop button) during suctioning. If pressure is "dumped" during suctioning, it may be necessary to re-pressurize the circuit (Reset button), and then start piston (Start/Stop button).

Weaning HFOV
Wean FIO_2 as tolerated to target SpO_2/PO_2
- Wean mPAW and ΔP - monitor SpO_2/PO_2 and CXR closely
  - Wean mPAW in 1-2 cmH_2O increments
  - Wean ΔP in 2-4 cmH_2O increments
- Consider extubating to NPPV or N-CPAP when:
  - mPAW = 7-9 cmH_2O
  - CXR is clear (or nearly clear)
  - FIO_2 < 30-40% (0.30 - 0.40)
  - Patient is noted to be breathing comfortably
  - Amplitude will usually be < 20

Note: Transition to conventional mechanical ventilation is not necessary, though it is common practice

HFOV Troubleshooting

(see manufacturer documentation for a more complete list)

Technical Troubleshooting

Oscillator stopped with no other alarms	• Ensure circuit has been re-pressurized (reset button) before starting piston • Ensure ΔP is > 6 cmH$_2$O • Ensure oscillator piston is centered
Unable to maintain Mean Airway Pressure	Check for leaks - • check all mushroom valves (cap diaphragm) • check water trap stopcock (ensure screwed in) • Check humidifier - with some therapeutic modalities, 1-way valves may be needed (e.g. iNO) • Check ET Tube Check bias flow rate - may be insufficient
Mean Airway Pressure not maintaining at desired value	• Pt may be spontaneously breathing (consider increasing sedation, use of a paralytic)
Will not Meet Circuit Calibration	• Check for leaks • Ensure adequate flowmeter setting
Low Pressure alarm	• Consider any break in circuit • Check mushroom valves, replace if necessary

Clinical Troubleshooting and Considerations

Increasing Respiratory Acidosis	- Decreased ET Tube diameter - Mucous plug - Pulmonary edema - Decreased Power or Amplitude settings - Decrease IT < 33% - Decreased Compliance - Increased Hertz
Patient Transport	- Avoid transport if possible - perform procedures and tests at bedside **If necessary**: - Clamp ET Tube with piston stopped, but HFOV on (circuit remains pressurized) - Bag pt with self-inflating manual resuscitator with PEEP valve (approximate mPAW from HFOV settings and bag with small, rapid breaths) - Unclamp ET tube and provide high quality ventilations - Strongly consider setting up an oscillator at destination—or a high PEEP strategy to maintain recruitment of lungs
Chest Wiggle Decreased	- ET tube moved or obstructed - Pneumothorax (unilateral ↓) - ET tube right mainstem (↓ wiggle on left side)
Increased mPaw, amplitude	- ET Tube obstruction (mucous) - Secretions - Bronchospasm - Rule out tension pneumothorax
Hypotension ↑ **CVP**	- Consider pulmonary overdistension

Modes 3-61

4 ASSESSMENT

Assessing Respiratory Distress.......................... 4-2
  Troubleshooting the Patient 4-4
  Troubleshooting the Ventilator..................... 4-5

Patient-Ventilator Assessment
  Considerations for Patient Assessment 4-6
  Considerations for Ventilator Assessment.... 4-7
  Acid-Base Values... 4-9
  Oxygenation.. 4-10
  Ventilation 4-11
  Ventilation Mechanics 4-12
    Static Compliance (Cstat) 4-13
    Dynamic Compliance (Cdyn) 4-13
    Airway Resistance (Raw) 4-14

Troubleshooting
See also Graphics Chapter
  Changes in V_T... 4-16
  Changes in Rate 4-17
  Changes in PIP 4-18
  Changes in PEEP 4-19
  Other Troubleshooting................................. 4-20
  Asynchrony 4-21

Assessment

Assessing Respiratory Distress on the Ventilator

Is the patient unstable? (rapidly assess)
- Diminished or unilateral chest movement
- Breath sounds decreased or absent
- Deteriorating vital signs (esp. bradycardia)

Yes to Any → **Patient is Unstable**

Disconnect from Ventilator
Provide manual ventilation (100% O_2)

→ Rapid Improvement
→ No Improvement

No to All → **Patient is Stable**
- Assess patient (pg 4-6)
- Analyze ventilator (pg 4-7)

next page

Ventilator Issue (see also pg 4-4)	
Analyze ventilator malfunction	• Perform vent and circuit checks (leak test, sensor tests, water in circuit, etc.) • If in doubt, trade device out
Inadequate or inappropriate settings	*More likely after initiation of vent or change in settings/mode* • Verify mode and settings are appropriate • Verify alarms are set properly (especially ones that limit parameters)

Patient Issue (see also pg 4-5)

If hypotension or bradycardia, consider life-threatening causes (tension pneumothorax, PE, cardiac event)

Increased resistance to bagging

Pass suction catheter:

- If difficult: ET tube blocked (suction), right mainstem (withdraw), kinked (reposition tube/head), cuff herniation (deflate)
- If not difficult: assess for tension pneumothorax, consider other causes (bronchospasm, etc.)

Normal resistance to bagging

- Perform assessment of patient in context of disease/disorder and clinical condition

Decreased/no resistance to bagging

- Consider cuff leak/extubation

Attempt to identify/reverse causes

Unsuccessful

Perform further systematic patient assessment, as indicated:
  Patient interview (yes/no questions)
  ECG, cardiac labs
  Capnography waveforms
  Vent alarm history
  Acid-base balance
  Respiratory mechanics (PIP, Pplat, etc.)
  Chest imaging

Consider trial of sedation/NMBA
If improvement, consider: delirium, pain, shock, hypercapnia/hypoxemia, etc.

Troubleshooting the Patient

Assess for:

Artificial Airway Patency	• Attempt to pass suction catheter • Cautiously consider instilling normal saline • Check for kinks/biting of ET tube
Endotracheal tube	• Placement Use ETCO$_2$, chest rise/auscultation. Do not reply solely on depth marking • Too deep: right mainstem • Too shallow: partial extubation • Improper placement: esophagus
Tracheostomy tube	• Placement Use ETCO$_2$, chest rise/auscultation • Check for subcutaneous emphysema (crepitus): malplaced in soft tissue (remove!)
Cuff Issues	• Cuff leak • Check integrity of cuff (measure pressure via pilot balloon) • Cuff balloon ruptured: won't inflate • Cuff balloon herniated: suction catheter may not pass easily
Tension pneumothorax	• Sudden ↑ in PIP, unilateral chest rise • Requires immediate decompression • Avoid positive pressure until resolved (may worsen)
Synchrony	• Analyze patient effort against ventilator's response (look at patient, check waveforms, etc.) • Is sedation level appropriate (assess pain, anxiety, oxygen consumption)
Bronchospasm	• Wheezing on auscultation? • Treat with SABAs

Troubleshooting the Ventilator

If any doubt about the ventilator, the patient must be taken off the ventilator and manually ventilated in order to isolate patient problems from ventilator issues.

Synchrony	Verify mode and parameters are appropriate for patient: • Trigger/Sensitivity (too sensitive, not sensitive enough) • Inappropriate Support (too much, too little) • Inadequate FiO_2 (hypoxemia)
Ventilator Leaks	• Check for leak/disconnect (patient and ventilator side)
Ventilator Obstructions	• Check ventilator filters and tubing for water • Check HME patency (secretions, water) • Verify exhalation valve is working (particularly when administering nebulized drugs) • If inline suction, verify suction catheter is in appropriate position in sheath (not obstructing ET Tube)

If any doubt about ventilator function exists, attempt to briefly troubleshoot. If the problem persists, strong consideration should be given to swapping out for a new ventilator.

Assessment

Considerations for Patient Assessment

Assess current parameters while trending for changes

Assess	Considerations
Appearance	• From bedside: Does patient appear comfortable? Any evidence of respiratory distress, anxiety, pain?
Auscultation	• Auscultate neck (listen for leak) • Auscultate all accessible lung fields - listen through inspiratory and expiratory phase of breath • Auscultate abdomen if any doubt of ET Tube placement
Sedation/LOC	• Check sedation level, paralytic? • Level of consciousness within context of sedation?
Vital Signs	• Check bedside monitor. Consider the impact of vent settings on BP, $ETCO_2$, SpO_2, etc.
Tubes/Lines	• Visually confirm presence of any tubes/lines and status of each (arterial line, central line, pulmonary artery catheter, chest tubes, bladder catheter)
Skin Integrity	• Verify skin integrity around artificial airways, finger probe, etc. • Any changes (redness, breakdown) should be documented and reported per policy • Place skin barriers and/or alter equipment
Other	• Verify head of patient 30-degrees or above (unless contraindicated) • Secretions: suction if indication, note quantity and characteristics of sputum

Considerations for Ventilator Assessment

Assess current parameters while trending for changes

Assess	Considerations
Verify orders	• Ensure settings consistent with current orders/protocols • Have appropriate changes been documented and communicated?
Mode	• Are mode and settings appropriate for the patient's current clinical condition?
Trigger (Sensitivity)	• Flow or pressure (or neural)? • Is patient triggering? • Is patient able to trigger, when desired (a negative pressure deflection in graphic should trigger a breath)? • Is ventilator triggering with no patient input (auto-triggering)?
Volumes	• Check V_T, minute ventilation • If volume mode, does delivered V_T equal return V_T ($V_{TI} = V_{TE}$) - if not: leak? air-trapping?
Pressures	• Check PIP, PEEP, CPAP, PS • Perform inspiratory hold (P_{plat}) • Perform expiratory hold (auto PEEP) • Calculate driving pressure (see pg 6-22)
Rate	• Does the patient have a spontaneous respiratory drive? If not, is this due to settings, sedation, underlying condition? Is it intentional?
Oxygen	• Ensure % appropriate to clinical condition • Consider ability to wean
Alarms	• Verify alarms are set and functioning and appropriate to the patient's condition • Ensure adequate backup settings • Verify volume is appropriate

Humidity	• If HME: clear of secretions? Change as indicated (~48-hrs to 1 wk)* • Humidifier: verify temperature (set, measured), water level, rainout in circuit
Synchrony	• Review ventilator graphics • Watch patient and ventilator. Does vent respond appropriately to patient activity (trigger, cycle, etc.)?

Equipment	• Check artificial airway
	   • ET tube: position, depth, tube tension
	   • Trach tube: position, tension on tube
	   • Check cuff pressures
	   • Check skin integrity
	 • Check circuit
	   • Position (avoid drainage back to the patient, if gravity-dependent area, consider water trap or change position)
	   • Clean: avoid routine circuit changes (breaking circuit increases risk of infection), but change if visibly soiled
	   • If heated wire circuit, verify appropriate temperature
	   • Avoid anything straining circuit

Safety	• Verify ventilator is connected to a red emergency outlet (accesses generator power in case of power loss)
	 • Ensure a manual resuscitator with mask (BVM) is at the bedside, flowmeter, PEEP valve if indicated (ideally, BVM is connected to flowmeter).
	   • If total laryngectomy, ensure pediatric mask (for use over stoma) is available.
	   • If tracheostomy, ensure obturator and spare trach tube is available
	 • Ensure suction equipment is connected, functional, and appropriate pressure

BVM = Bag-Valve Mask
* AARC Evidence-Based Guidelines

Acid-Base Values

A-V difference (right-most column) helps estimate the difference between an arterial sample and a venous sample.

Parameter	Arterial (ABG)		Venous* (peripheral VBG)		A-V Difference
	Norm	Range	Norm	Range	Average
pH units	pHa 7.40	7.35-7.45	pH$\bar{v}$ 7.36	7.31-7.41	0.04
PCO_2 mmHg	PaCO_2 40	35-45	P$\bar{v}CO_2$ 46	40-50	6
PO_2 (Room Air) mmHg	PaO_2 100	80-100	P$\bar{v}O_2$ 40	30-50	55
O_2 Sat %	SaO_2 97	95-100	S$\bar{v}O_2$ 75	68-77	22
HCO_3^- mEq/L	24	22-26	24	23-27	1
TCO_2** mEq/L	25	23-27	25	23-27	none
BE mEq/L	0	+/- 2	0	+/- 2	none
O_2 content mL/dL	CaO_2 20	15-24	C$\bar{v}O_2$ 15	12-15	> 2

* Venous values depend on where the sample was drawn from. The above chart lists peripheral values. When analyzing a sample from a central line (CVP) or pulmonary artery (PA) catheter:
(compared to ABG)

pH	▼ 0.03 - 0.05
PCO_2	▲ 3-8
HCO_3^-	▲ 2-3

Peripheral values may vary if peripheral circulation is compromised
All values may vary if hypotension, shock, or extreme acid-base imbalance

** TCO_2 is more a reflection of HCO_3^- than CO_2 [TCO_2 = HCO_3^- + 0.03(PCO_2)]

Assessment

Oxygenation Assessment

Oxygenation at the Lungs (external respiration)		Oxygenation at the Tissues (internal respiration)	
Measure	Clinically Acceptable Range*	Measure	Clinically Acceptable Range*
Adequacy			
PaO_2*	80-100 mmHg (< 60 concerning)	$P\bar{v}O_2$	35-42 mmHg
CaO_2	15-24 mL/dL	$C\bar{v}O_2$	12-15 mL/dL
SaO_2	> 92-95%	$S\bar{v}O_2$	60-80%
SpO_2	> 92-95%	$C(a-\bar{v})O_2$	4.5-5.0 mL/dL
Efficiency			
$P(A-a)O_2$	10-25 mmHg (room air) 30-50 mmHg (FiO_2 1.0)	$O2_{ER}$	25%
		$\dot{V}O_2$	200-250 mL/min
		$\dot{D}O_2$	750 - 1000 mL/min
P/F ratio (PaO_2/FiO_2)	> 300 (< 200 concerning)	VQI	0.8
S/F ratio (SpO_2/FiO_2)	~ P/F ratio		
Oxygenation Index	< 25		

*These ranges are not absolutes, but are meant to guide clinical assessment within the context of disease/disorder

Ventilation Assessment

Value	Range	Clinical Notes
Adequacy		
Minute Ventilation	5-10 L/min	Verify if caused by underlying patient condition or ventilator settings (calculate VT based on IBW, rate)
$PaCO_2$	35-45 torr	Interpret in context of pH (and patient's baseline)
$ETCO_2$	35-43 torr	Continuous monitoring is preferred
Efficiency		
V_{Dphys}	⅓ $\dot{V}_E$	Physiologic deadspace is the sum of anatomic and alveolar deadspace
V_D/V_T	0.33-0.45	An increase suggests abnormal gas exchange Difficult to estimate at bedside

Changes in Ventilation
Assess within the context of vent mode/settings, sedation, etc.

Hyperventilation (respiratory alkalosis)
- Excessive ventilator settings
- Metabolic acidosis (most common cause)
- Hypoxemia
- Pain
- Anxiety
- Underlying condition (brain injury, etc.)

Hypoventilation (respiratory acidosis)
- Inadequate ventilator settings
- Sedation/neuromuscular blockade (paralytics)
- Respiratory muscle weakness
- Underlying condition (respiratory center depression, etc.)
- Trauma

Assessment

Ventilation Mechanics Assessment

See specific causes of changes on following pages

Value	Range	Clinical Notes
Load		
Dynamic Compliance	40-60 mL/cmH$_2$O	
Static Compliance	70-100 mL/cmH$_2$O	
Airway Resistance	0.5-2.5 cmH$_2$O/L/sec	Artificial airway: 4-8 cmH$_2$O/L/sec
RSBI (f/VT)	less than 100-105	Evaluate readiness to extubate (on minimal settings) - see pg 11-19 for important clinical notes
Respiratory Drive		
P0.1	less than 2 cmH$_2$O	Negative pressure measured 100 ms after inspiratory effort initiation correlates with the central respiratory drive*
Respiratory Muscle Strength		
Vital Capacity	60-80 mL/kg	< 30 mL/kg is concerning
PImax MIP, NIF	More negative than -60 to -80 cmH$_2$O	more positive than -20 to -30 on a ventilator is concerning

* Beloncle F, Piquilloud L, Oliver P, Vuillermoz A, Yvin E, Mercat A, Richard J. Accuracy of P0.1 measurements performed by ICU ventilators: A bench study. Annals of Intens Care 2019;9(104).

Changes in Static Compliance (Cstat)

> Strategies for improving Cstat is to preferably address the underlying cause (reverse atelectasis, treat auto-PEEP, etc.), but when not possible, implement strategies to compensate (see Disease/Disorder chapter)

Decreased Cstat
- When acute, may be a sign that underlying condition is worsening, or something else is wrong
- Air trapping (auto-PEEP)
- Disease/disorder (ARDS, atelectasis, consolidation, fibrosis, pneumothorax, pleural effusion)
- Endotracheal tube issue (tube advanced too far into bronchus)
- Abdominal pressures (ascites, obesity, pregnancy, etc.)
- Physical (kyphoscoliosis, obesity, pectus excavatum, etc.)

Increased Cstat
- When acute, may be a sign that underlying condition is improving
- COPD (especially emphysema)
- Flail chest
- Patient position change

Changes in Dynamic Compliance (Cdyn)

Dynamic compliance is dependent on static compliance (see above) and airway resistance (see next page)

Changes in Airway Resistance (Raw)
A decrease in Raw is considered an improvement

> Improving airway resistance is about identifying the cause(s) and managing those (see diseases/disorders)

Increased Raw
- **Airway Obstructions**
    - Artificial airway issue
      (small diameter, plugging, malplacement in soft tissue, kinking or biting if ET tube, in-line suction left in airway)
    - Condensation/secretions in circuit (rainout) or HME
    - Physical obstructions (secretions, mucosal edema, mucous plugs, foreign bodies, tumors)

- **Collapse of Airways**
    - Bronchoconstriction/spasm
    - Disease/disorder (asthma, bronchitis, COPD, pleural effusion, pneumothorax, etc.)
    - Tracheomalacia
    - Tumors

- **High flow** (causing turbulence)

Troubleshooting

The following pages contain troubleshooting considerations for clinical scenarios.
- Consider options in context of the patient's disease/disorder, clinical status, other pertinent findings (fluid status, infection, etc.)
- Not all problems are solvable (such as when related to some pathophysiology). When this is the case, the goal shifts to strategizing ways to compensate or provide sufficient support (optimizing oxygenation through positioning, for example)

For general considerations in optimizing oxygenation and ventilation, see Chapter 7 (Clinical Management)

Changes in Tidal Volume (VT)

> In pressure modes, tidal volume is a reflection of Raw and C. In volume modes, tidal volumes don't change (or at least by much). Some modes with a set VT use pressure limits as a safety mechanism, which could result in a lower-than-set VT as well.
>
> When expired tidal volume is lower than inspired tidal volume, consider the possibility of a leak or air-trapping.

Decreased VT
Inspired
- If volume mode: are breaths pressure-limiting due to change in Raw or C? Has setting been inadvertently changed?
- If pressure mode: increase in Raw (see pg 4-14) or decrease in C (see pg 4-13 for causes)

Expired
- If Expired VT is less than Inspired VT, consider presence of:
    - Vent circuit leak
    - Patient (active air leak, chest tube)
    - Air trapping (auto-PEEP)

Increased VT
- If volume mode: is there external flow being added to the circuit (nebulizer)? Has VT been inadvertently changed?
- If pressure mode: decrease in Raw or increase in C

Changes in Rate

> Rates should never decrease below a set rate, but usually can increase above that rate (unless pure CMV mode where a patient is locked out).
>
> A high rate has many causes. Treating the underlying cause, when possible and appropriate, is usually most helpful. Sedating to normalize the rate is an option, but in some situations the impact of this must be considered (increased metabolic needs, for example).

Decreased Rate

Set rate should not decrease unless:
- Setting is changed
- Ventilator malfunction
- Disconnect

Spontaneous/supported rate:
- Improvement in condition/support (PS, VS, for example)
- Sedation or paralytic started or increased

Increased Rate

Set rate should not increase unless:
- Setting is changed
- Ventilator malfunction

Spontaneous rate may increase in response to:
- Hypoxemia, or other causes of increased metabolic demand (fever, sepsis)
- Pain or anxiety (look at vital signs, patient)
- Auto-triggering (inappropriate trigger)
- Cardiogenic oscillations (HR triggered breath)
- Nebulizer flow causing triggers

Assessment

Changes in Inspiratory Pressure (PIP)

> In pressure modes, inspiratory pressure is set. In volume modes, inspiratory pressure varies in response to changes in Raw and C.
>
> Increases in PIP do not directly correlate with lung injury in all situations, which is why Cstat and ΔP should be monitored as well (better reflections of lung injury risk).
>
> Differentiate between transient changes (such as with coughing) and trended changes (change in patient condition)

Decreased PIP
- Changed settings
- Improving compliance or airway resistance will decrease PIP in volume modes
- Disconnect or leak (vent, circuit, cuff, chest tube, fistula)

Increased PIP
- Changed settings in pressure control
- Worsening compliance or airway resistance will increase PIP in volume modes - see pg 4-13 to 4-14
- Asynchrony (fighting the ventilator)
- Problem with exhalation valve

> **Checking for Leaks**
> 1. ***Check Patient***
>   Remove patient from ventilator and manually ventilate.
>   Listen to breath sounds over trachea.
>   ET tube cuff inflated?
>
> 2. ***Check Ventilator:***
>   Obstruct patient wye and manually cycle the ventilator.
>   If the high pressure alarm fails to activate (in volume modes), obstruct the patient circuit at various places starting at the ventilator and working distal to find the leak (until the alarm does not activate).

Changes in Positive End Expiratory Pressure (PEEP)

> PEEP should stay steady, or close to steady, at the set amount. Monitored PEEP that varies from the set PEEP is considered abnormal.

Decreased PEEP
- Changed settings
- Decreased expiratory flow
- Increased inspiratory flowrate

Increased PEEP
- Changed settings
- Increased expiratory flow
- Presence of air trapping (auto-PEEP)
- Patient-ventilatory asynchrony

Other Troubleshooting

> After brief troubleshooting, if any doubt, consider pulling the ventilator from service

Gas Supply Alert
- Verify gas hoses are connected correctly to 50 PSI
- Verify integrity of hoses (not under a bed wheel, etc.)
- Consider running calibration test
- Verify zone valve hasn't been altered
- If gas supply failure, consider alternative gas by cylinder (backfeed 50 PSI if able)
- FIO_2 error: analyzer may be uncalibrated, defective, or disconnected.

Power Loss
- Ensure power switch hasn't been inadvertently switched off
- Ensure ventilator plugged in (red outlet)

Ventilator Inoperative
- Remove patient from ventilator, reset, perform pre-use check to verify function

Patient-Ventilator Asynchrony
See Ch 5 for Graphics related to Asynchrony
See Ch 7 for Detailed Causes and Strategies

> Our goal, whenever possible, is to optimize ventilator settings to be in synch with (responsive to) the patient's needs. When clinical goals override this ability, higher levels of sedation may be necessary.

Potential Causes
- Artificial Airway Issues (size, biting, secretions)
- Auto-PEEP (disease, ventilator settings)
- Expiratory Valves
- Humidifiers (HME or heated humidity)
- Trigger sensitivity (auto-, reverse-, or missed)
- Mode asynchrony (inadequate, excessive support)
- Flow asynchrony
- Cycle asynchrony

5 Graphics

Explanations/Introduction..............................5-3

Types of Graphics
Scalars
Pressure-Time...5-4
Volume-Time..5-7
Flow-Time 5-9
Loops
Pressure-Volume...5-11
Flow-Volume..5-14

Normal Graphics
Scalars...5-16
Loops 5-22

Abnormal Graphics
(by waveform)
Scalars...5-26
Loops 5-30
(by problem)
Patient
Air-Trapping (auto-PEEP)...............................5-36
Airway Resistance Changes...........................5-38
Compliance Changes....................................5-41
Active Exhalation..5-43
Partial Obstruction 5-44
Ventilator
Overdistension...5-45
Leaks 5-46
Rate (Cycle) Asynchrony...............................5-48
Flow Asynchrony (Flow Starvation)...............5-49
Trigger Asynchrony......................................5-50

Other Applications 5-52

What are Graphics?

Graphics, sometimes also called "waveform graphics," or simply by its type. "loops" or "scalars" provide valuable information about the interaction of the ventilator with the patient.

Scalars are two-dimensional. The x-axis is always *time*, and the Y axis is either *flow, pressure, or volume*.

Loops display the relationship between any two of the non-time parameters: *flow, pressure, and volume*.

Indications

Graphics should be considered at each patient-ventilator assessment, paying specific attention to:
- Clinical progression (compliance and resistance changes)
- Response to therapies (bronchodilators, etc.)
- Patient-Ventilator synchrony
- Parameter optimization
- Troubleshooting (auto-PEEP, secretions, etc.)

Clinical Notes

Initial analysis involves identifying the scale, mode, and parameters so that normal versus abnormal can be considered
This chapter contains representations. In clinical care graphics vary widely by situation, multiple issues, etc.
The goal in understanding and interpreting graphics is not to memorize shapes, but rather to understand how they are created and how they are affected by variables.

Graphics

Types Of Graphic Waveforms

> **Scalars** – Graphic displays of **pressure, volume,** and **flow** over time.
> **Loops** – Graphic displays of two parameters (**Pressure and Volume** or **Flow and Volume**) on a horizontal (x) axis and a vertical (y) axis. Time is not depicted on loops.

Scalars

Pressure-Time Scalar

Spontaneous breath:

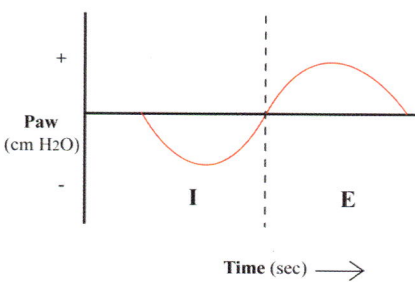

Ventilator breath:

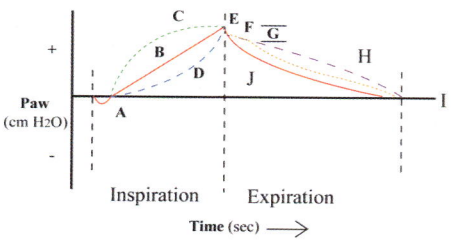

Pressure-Time Key (from diagram on previous page)

A	Deflection below the baseline indicates a patient-trigger (effort). If an assisted breath, this should be followed by a positive waveform (breath). A breath with no negative deflection is a ventilator-triggered breath The greater the depth and time below baseline, the greater the patient effort required to trigger the ventilator. Flow-triggering (flow-by) will eliminate most patient effort, resulting in less negative deflection.
B	Square wave inspiratory flow pattern The steeper the slope, the greater the $\dot{V}_I$
C	Decelerating inspiratory flow pattern
D	Sine wave inspiratory flow pattern

E	Peak inspiratory pressure (Ppeak)
	    Ppeak may rise to a plateau when a breath is pressure-controlled (limited) or pressure-supported. This Ppeak pressure plateau is not to be confused with Pplat.
	    Used with Cdyn

F	Plateau pressure (Pplat)
	    Results from an inspiratory hold
	    Used to calculate Cstat

G	Ppeak − Pplat = Raw (Raw is flow dependent) Pressure required to overcome resistance of airway and ET tube.

H	Expiratory retard
	    Similar to pursed-lip breathing
	    May be patient-induced (e.g., COPD) or ventilator-induced (rarely done)

I	Baseline pressure (beginning and end-expiratory pressure)
	    ZEEP – zero (atmospheric)
	    PEEP – positive (above zero)
	    NEEP – negative (below zero)
	Failure of the pressure curve to return to the set baseline pressure before the next inspiration = inadequate TE and may result in air-trapping

J	Area under the entire curve, including any PEEP, is ≈ average $\overline{Paw}$

Clinical Applications of Pressure-Time Scalar

Patient
- Air-trapping (auto-PEEP)
- Airway obstruction
- Active exhalation
- Bronchodilator response
- Respiratory mechanics (C + Raw)

Ventilator
- Breath type (mode)
- Identifying and monitoring peak pressures
- Measure plateau pressure (during an inspiratory hold)
- Identifying and monitoring PEEP or CPAP
- Identifying and monitoring T_I, T_E, I:E

Patient-Ventilator Interactions
- Asynchrony
- Triggering effort

Volume-Time Scalar

Spontaneous breath:

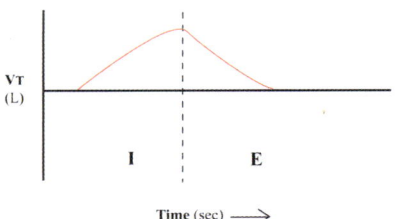

Ventilator breath:

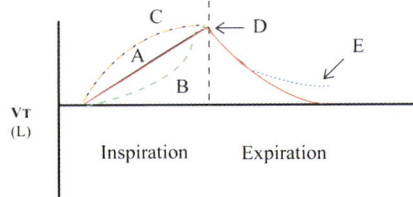

A	Square wave inspiratory flow pattern
B	Sine wave inspiratory flow pattern
C	Decelerating inspiratory flow pattern (or pressure-supported breath)
D	Inspiratory V_T (a plateau at this peak of the curve may indicate pressure-controlled or supported breath)
E	An exhalation curve that does not return to baseline may indicate leak or air-trapping

Clinical Applications of Volume-Time Scalar

Patient
- Air-trapping (auto-PEEP)
- Active exhalation

Ventilator
- Breath type (mode)
- Identifying and monitoring V_T, flow
- Identify potential leaks

Patient-Ventilator Interactions
- Asynchrony

Flow-Time Scalar

Spontaneous breath:

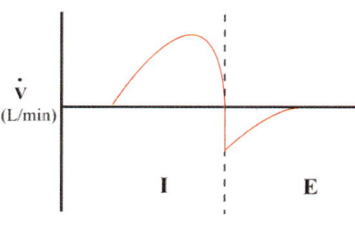

Ventilator breaths:

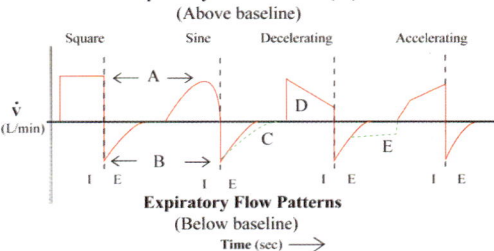

A	Peak inspiratory flow (set $\dot{V}_I$)
B	Peak expiratory flow
C	Expiratory retard— Increased resistance to expiratory flow (see H under pressure-time curve)
B/C	Evaluation of response to bronchodilator administration

continued next page

D	Pressure-control and supported breaths have a decelerating flow pattern
E	Expiratory flow patterns have one basic shape and should return to baseline(zero flow) indicating a complete exhalation
	Expiratory flow that does not return to zero prior to the next inspiration, indicates inadequate T_E, resulting in air-trapping and auto-PEEP (most modes)
	(The higher the end-expiratory flow, the greater the auto-PEEP)
	An expiratory flow that returns to above the baseline indicates a leak during flow-by.

Clinical Applications of Flow-Time Scalar
Patient
- Air-trapping (auto-PEEP)
- Active exhalation
- Airway obstruction
- Response to bronchodilator administration
- Respiratory mechanics (compliance and resistance)

Ventilator
- Breath type (mode)
- Identifying and monitoring flow issues (waveform shape, starvation in volume, inspiratory flow)
- Identify potential leaks
- Analyzing and adjusting rise of pressure time (pressure control)

Patient-Ventilator Interactions
- Asynchrony
- Triggering effort

Loops

Pressure-Volume Loop

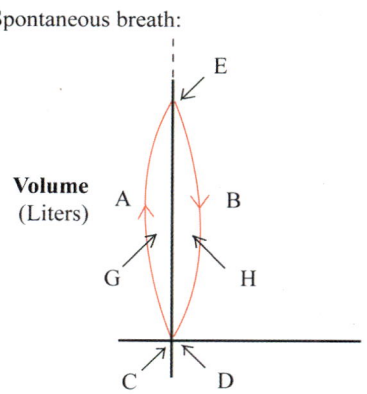

Spontaneous breath:

Ventilator Breath (Volume Ventilation)

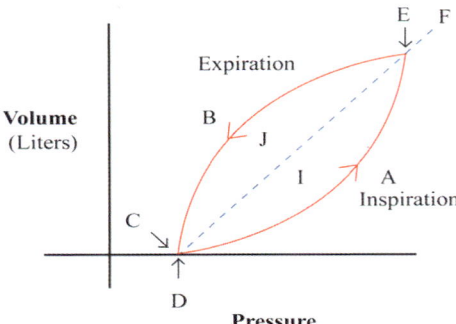

A	Inspiratory curve (upward)

B	Expiratory curve (downward)
	    Positive pressure breaths go counter-clockwise (arrows)
	    Spontaneous pressure breaths go clockwise (not shown)

C	The bottom point of the loop: Inspiration begins and expiration ends
D	Point on pressure axis where inspiration (I) begins and expiration (E) ends (indicates end-expiratory pressure level)

E	The upper point of the loop:
	    1) Inspiration ends and expiration begins
	    2) Point of maximal pressure and volume
	    3) Dynamic compliance ($\Delta V/\Delta P$)

F	The imaginary (dashed) line between the 2 points (C & E), (begin I & end I) depicts the slope of the loop. The slope is a reflection of the patient's dynamic compliance ($\Delta V/\Delta P$)
G	The area to the left of the vertical line represents patient inspiratory WOB (inspiratory resistance)
H	The area to the right of the vertical axis represents patient expiratory WOB (expiratory resistance)

I	The area of the curve to the right of the slope line depicts the ventilator WOB (amount of pressure needed to deliver a certain volume) required to overcome Raw. (↑ area = ↑ work)
J	The area of the curve to the left of the slope line depicts the WOB required to overcome C_{RS}
	Total WOB = area I and area J (↑ area = ↑ work)

Note: These areas show only the mechanical WOB by the ventilator and are only accurate if the patient is not contributing any WOB. Patient WOB can be measured indirectly by plotting the esophageal pressure.

Clinical Applications

Patient	Ventilator	Patient-Ventilator Interaction
• Airway obstruction • Active exhalation • Bronchodilator response • Lung over-distension • Respiratory mechanics • (Cdyn + Raw) • WOB	• Adjusting pressure support levels • Flow starvation (volume modes) • Leaks	• Triggering effort

Flow-Volume Loop

Spontaneous breath:

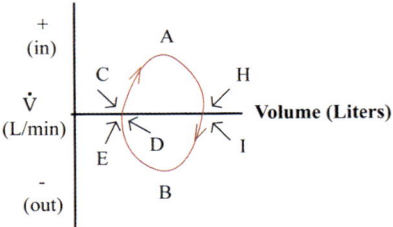

Ventilator breath:
(Volume Ventilation)

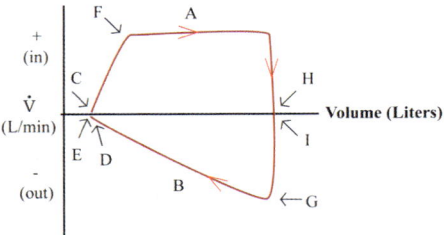

A	Inspiratory curve (above the horizontal axis) On the ventilator breath, the shape of the inspiratory curve will reflect the flow pattern set on the ventilator.
B	Expiratory curve (below the horizontal axis) The shape of the expiratory curve will reflect patient exhalation (usually passive).
C	Begin inspiration
D	End expiration
E	Point on volume axis where I begins and E ends. This indicates end-expiratory pressure level. Note: C, D, and E should all be the same point. (See abnormal waveforms if not)

F	Peak inspiratory flow rate ($\dot{V}_I$)
G	Peak expiratory flow rate
H	Point on volume axis of maximum V_T and end inspiration (flow rate 0)
I	Begin expiration Note: H and I should be the same point. (See abnormal waveforms if not)

* **Note**:

Pulmonary function flow-volume loops (depicting FVC) traditionally display the inspiratory curve <u>below</u> the horizontal axis and expiration above the axis.

Ventilator flow-volume loops (depicting V_T) most commonly display the inspiratory curve <u>above</u> the horizontal axis and expiration below the axis (to maintain consistency with scalars).

There is, however, no set convention and some ventilators will display the loops like pulmonary function loops. When reading flow-volume loops be certain to properly identify the orientation.

This book will display all loops with the inspiratory curve <u>above</u> the axis.

Clinical Applications

Patient	Ventilator	Pt-Vent Interaction
• Air-trapping (auto-PEEP) • Airway obstruction • Airway resistance changes • Active exhalation • Bronchodilator response	• Inspiratory flow • Expiratory flow • Flow starvation (volume modes) • V_T • Leaks • Water and secretions buildup	• Asynchrony

Normal Graphic Waveforms by Waveform Type

Scalars: Pressure-Time

The pressure-time scalar is the best way to identify a patient-triggered breath as a deflection below the baseline. The depth of deflection and the amount of time below baseline reflect patient effort. Flow-triggering usually eliminates this patient effort.

Spontaneous Ventilation

During inspiration, pressure is a negative deflection. During expiration, pressure is a positive deflection

Pressures are usually lower than with ventilator breaths

I to E is patient-cycled

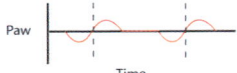

Volume Ventilation – Assist/Control (constant or square flow)

The pressure curve shows a linear rise to Ppeak

Ppeak is dependent on V_T, $\dot{V}_I$, PEEP, C, and Raw

I to E is volume-cycled

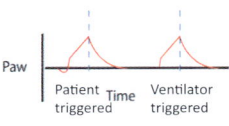

Volume Ventilation – Assist/Control (decelerating flow)

Same as square flow (above), except that the upward slope to Ppeak is usually more curved

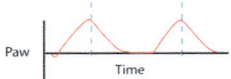

Volume - SIMV (square flow)

A combination of assisted and spontaneous ventilation

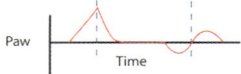

Pressure Ventilation – Assist/Control

The pressure curve shows an immediate rise to Ppeak (set pressure), which is maintained during the entire inspiratory phase. The speed (slope) in which set pressure is reached is dependent on the ventilator (rise time). Patient C and Raw generally do not affect the shape of the waveform.

I to E is time-cycled (T_I is constant)

Ppeak = Pplat, assuming there is zero flow at end-inspiration

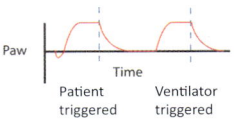

Pressure Support

Similar to Pressure A/C (above), but:
1. Ppeak is usually lower (unless PSmax is set)
2. Every breath is an assisted breath
3. I to E is flow-cycled (T_I may vary between breaths)

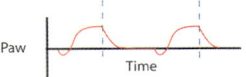

Graphics

Scalars: Volume-Time

Spontaneous Ventilation

The volume achieved is dependent on patient effort, C, and Raw. The rise to achieved volume is sinusoidal.
I to E is patient-cycled

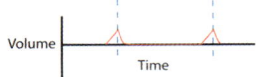

Volume Ventilation – Assist/Control
(constant or square flow)

The volume delivered is set
The rise to delivered V_T is linear.
I to E is volume-cycled.

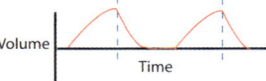

Patient triggered · Time · Ventilator triggered

Volume Ventilation – Assist/Control
(decelerating flow)

Same as square flow (above), except that the rise to delivered V_T is usually more curved

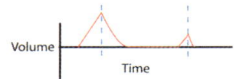

Volume-SIMV
(constant or square flow)

A combination of assisted and spontaneous ventilation.

Pressure Ventilation – Assist/Control

The volume delivered is determined by the set pressure level, C, and Raw of the lungs
The rise to deliver the V_T is initially rapid, followed by a decrease, then a plateau
I to E is time-cycled (T_I is constant)

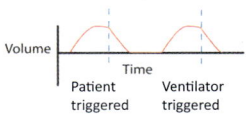

Pressure Support

Similar to PV (above), but:
1. The delivered volume (plateau) is usually lower
2. The delivered volume is dependent on:
   - Set pressure support
   - Patient effort, compliance, and resistance
3. Every breath is supported
4. I to E is flow-cycled (T_I may vary between breaths)

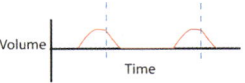

Scalars: Flow-Time

Spontaneous Ventilation

The inspiratory curve is sinusoidal in shape, but highly variable, depending on patient effort. Peak flows are generally much lower than with ventilator breaths. I to E is patient-cycled

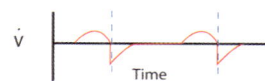

Volume Ventilation – Assist/Control (constant or square flow)

Flow reaches a maximum at the beginning of I and continues at that maximum during the entire inspiratory phase. I to E is volume-cycled.

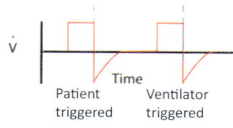

Volume Ventilation – Assist/Control (decelerating flow)

Same as square flow (above), except that inspiratory flow decelerates during the inspiratory phase. Since I to E is volume-cycled, flow may or may not reach zero before end-inspiration.

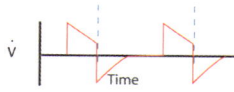

SIMV - Volume

A combination of assisted and spontaneous ventilation.

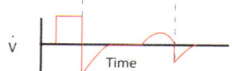

Pressure Ventilation – Assist/Control

Inspiratory flow reaches a maximum at the beginning of I and then decelerates during the inspiratory phase. Flow is variable depending on patient's C and Raw.
I to E is time-cycled (hence T_I is constant). Since I to E is time-cycled, flow may or may not reach zero before end-inspiration. If flow does not reach zero, T_I may be too short.

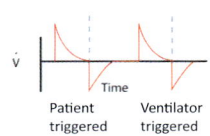

Patient triggered   Ventilator triggered

Pressure Support

Inspiratory flow reaches a maximum at the beginning of I and then decelerates during the inspiratory phase. Flow is 0variable depending on patient's C and Raw. Every breath is an assisted breath.
I to E is flow-cycled (T_I may vary between breaths). I terminates when $\dot{V}_I$ decreases to a ventilator determined flow (usually 25% of peak flow) (flow never reaches zero)

Clinical note: the Flow-Time waveform is the best way to identify a PS breath.

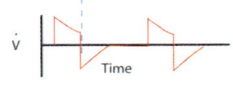

Loops: Pressure-Volume

Spontaneous Ventilation

The loop is clockwise in spontaneous breathing. The inspiratory curve is generally to the left of baseline pressure (vertical axis) due to negative pressure during inspiration. The expiratory curve is generally to the right of the baseline pressure due to positive expiratory pressure. The area to the left of the vertical axis represents patient inspiratory WOB (inspiratory resistance). The area to the right of the vertical axis represents patient expiratory WOB (expiratory resistance).

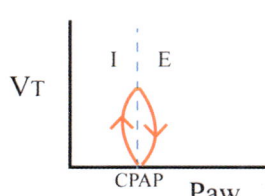

Volume Ventilation – Assist/Control (constant or square flow)

The loop is counter-clockwise with ventilator breaths During an assisted breath, the inspiratory area to the left of the vertical axis represents the patient WOB required to initiate inspiration. The greater the area, the greater the WOB imposed by the ventilator.

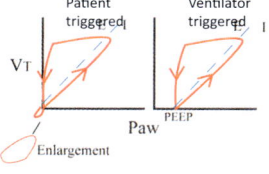

Volume Ventilation – Assist/Control (decelerating flow)

Same as square flow (above), except the inspiratory portion is more curved

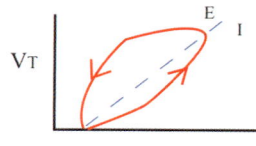

SIMV - Volume
(constant or square flow)

A combination of spontaneous and assisted ventilations

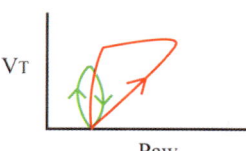

Pressure Ventilation – Assist/Control

The set pressure is reached quickly before the volume has a chance to rise.

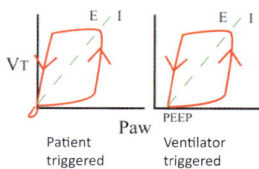

Pressure Support

Similar to PV, except:
1. Pressure and volume are usually less
2. Each breath is supported

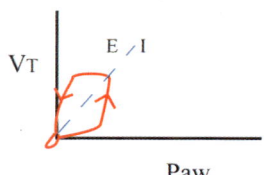

Loops: Flow-Volume

Spontaneous Ventilation

The loop is usually quite circular due to the natural sinusoidal flow rates

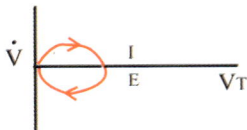

Volume Ventilation – Assist/Control (constant or square flow)

Flow reaches a maximum at the beginning of I and continues at that maximum during the entire inspiratory phase. V_T is peaked as the flow switches from positive to negative (I to E).

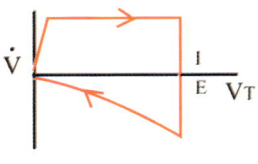

Volume Ventilation – Assist/Control (decelerating flow)

Same as square flow (above), except inspiratory flow decelerates during the inspiratory phase

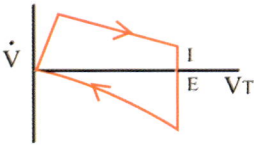

SIMV - Volume (constant or square flow)

A combination of spontaneous and assisted ventilations

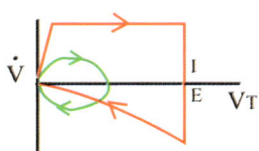

Pressure Ventilation – Assist/Control

Flow reaches a maximum at the beginning of I and then decelerates during the inspiratory phase. VT is peaked as the flow switches from positive to negative (I to E).

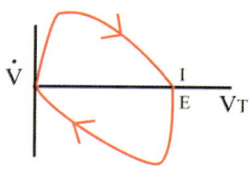

Pressure Support

Similar to PV, except:
1. Flow and volume are usually less
2. The inspiratory phase is terminated when $\dot{V}_i$ decreases to a ventilator determined flow (usually 25% of peak flow) (never reaches zero)
3. Each breath is supported

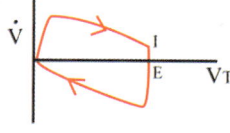

Abnormal Graphics by Waveform Type

For the description of a particular graph, turn to the Abnormal Graphic Waveform By Problem section and proceed to the particular problem.

Examples given in volume ventilation. Because PIP is set in pressure modes, changes are less likely to impact pressure graphics.

Abnormal Scalars: Pressure-Time

Air-trapping (auto-PEEP)

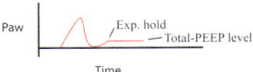

Airway Resistance (worsening)

Increases the difference between PIP and Pplat (Pplat remains steady). The dashed line is Pplat

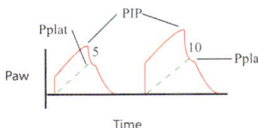

Compliance (worsening)

Increases PIP and Pplat but Raw (PIP - Pplat) remains the same. The dashed line is Pplat.

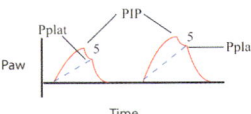

Leaks

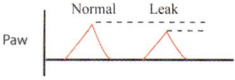

Rate (Cycle) Asynchrony

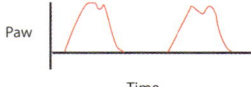

**Flow Asynchrony
(Flow Starvation)
 in Volume Ventilation**

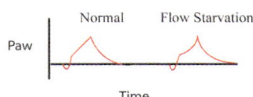

**Trigger Asynchrony
(Inappropriate Trigger)**

Mimics auto-PEEP triggering asynchrony

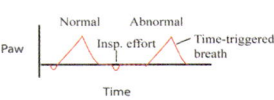

**Trigger Asynchrony
(Auto-PEEP)**

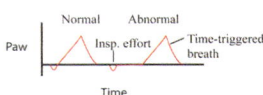

Graphics   5-27

Abnormal Scalars: Volume-Time

Air-trapping (auto-PEEP)
may look like a leak

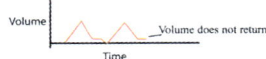

Airway Resistance (worsening)

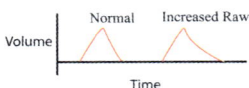

Excessive (Active) Exhalation

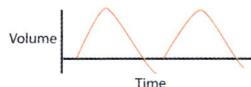

Leaks

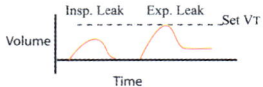

Abnormal Scalars: Flow-Time

Air-trapping (auto-PEEP)

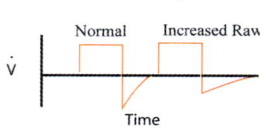

Airway Resistance (worsening)

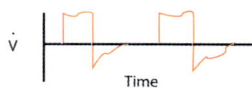

Partial Obstruction

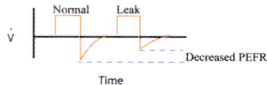

Leaks

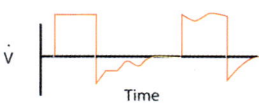

Rate (Cycle) Asynchrony

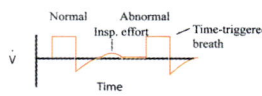

Trigger Asynchrony
(Inappropriate Sensitivity Setting)

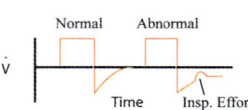

Trigger Asynchrony
(Auto-PEEP)

Graphics 5-29

Abnormal Loops: Pressure-Volume

Air-trapping (auto-PEEP)

Example: Volume Ventilation

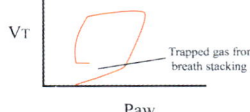

Airway Resistance Changes (Ventilator Breath)
Dashed lines depicts normal and solid line is ↑ Raw
Example: Volume Ventilation

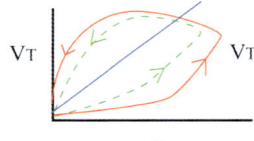

Airway Resistance Changes (Spontaneous Breath)
Dashed lines depicts normal and solid line is ↑ Raw

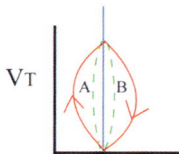

Compliance Changes

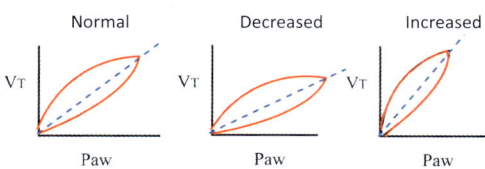

Excessive (Active) Exhalation

Example: Volume Ventilation

Partial Obstruction

Example: Volume Ventilation

Over-distension

Leaks

Example: Volume Ventilation

Rate (Cycle) Asynchrony

Example: Volume Ventilation

Graphics

Flow Asynchrony (Flow Starvation)

Example: Volume Ventilation

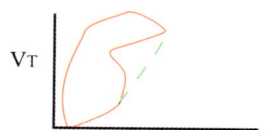

Trigger Asynchrony (Inappropriate Sensitivity Setting)

Example: Volume Ventilation

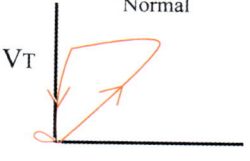

Abnormal Loops: Flow-Volume

All examples are Volume Ventilation

Air-trapping (auto-PEEP)

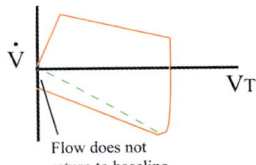

Flow does not return to baseline

Airway Resistance Changes

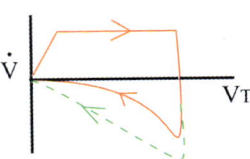

Excessive (Active) Exhalation

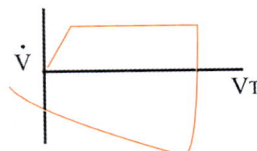

Partial Obstruction

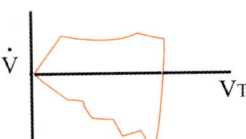

Leaks

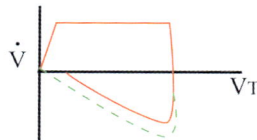

Rate (Cycle) Asynchrony

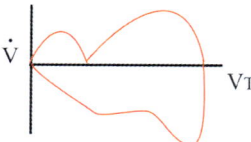

Abnormal Graphic Waveforms by Problem

Section Contents
Patient
    Air-trapping (auto-PEEP)
    Airway resistance changes
    Compliance changes
    Excessive exhalation
    Partial obstruction

Ventilator
    Over-distension
    Leaks

Patient-Ventilator Interaction
    Rate asynchrony
    Flow asynchrony
    Trigger asynchrony (inappropriate sensitivity setting)
    Trigger asynchrony (auto-PEEP)

All examples are in Volume Ventilation.

Air Trapping (auto-PEEP)
Causes and Strategies

- **Dynamic hyperinflation** (insufficient T_E for complete expiration) due to:
  1. Increased expiratory Raw (prolonged expiration)
  2. Decreased T_E (insufficient time before next breath)

  > T_E needs to be extended, which can be done conventionally by decreasing TI and/or decreasing the vent set rate

- **Early collapse of unstable alveoli during expiration**
  (exhaled air is blocked from flowing out)

  > Stabilizing the alveoli is the priority. Using PEEP/CPAP may be considered as a trial.

Pressure-Time
Auto-PEEP can only be identified (and quantified) when an expiratory hold is employed. During the hold, baseline pressure line rises to the auto-PEEP level (depicting pressure still trapped in alveoli). If applied PEEP is employed, the expiratory hold baseline will rise to total PEEP (applied PEEP + auto-PEEP).

Clinical Note: Sufficient hold time must be employed to allow the pressure to reach a plateau, plus there must be no patient effort during the hold.

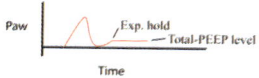

Volume-Time
Volume does not return to baseline (depicting volume still trapped in alveoli). The less the return, the greater the air-trapping. *Note*: this is the same curve as a leak —see Leak.

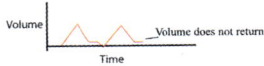

Flow-Time
Expiratory flow does not return to baseline (depicting flow still trapped in alveoli). The less the return, the greater the air-trapping. The dashed line depicts normal flow return to baseline.

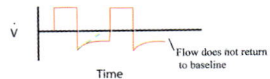

Pressure-Volume
Volume does not return to baseline (depicting volume still trapped in alveoli). The less the return, the greater the air-trapping.

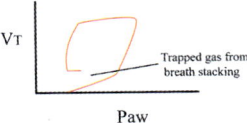

Flow-Volume
Expiratory flow does not return to baseline (depicting flow still trapped in alveoli). The less the return, the greater the air-trapping. The dashed line depicts normal flow return to baseline.

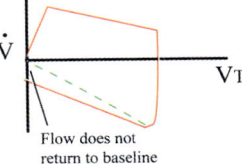

Graphics 5-37

Increased Airway Resistance
Causes and Strategies
- Bronchospasm
- Damp or blocked expiratory filter
- ET tube (small size, bitten, kinked, or partially obstructed)
- High inspiratory flow
- Secretion buildup (see also water/secretion problem)

> Address the underlying issue when possible. This can be as simple as administering a SABA for bronchospasm, suctioning secretions, exchanging with a larger ET tube, or it can be much more complex. Trial options and check for response.

Pressure-Time
Using an inspiratory pause (hold), the difference between Ppeak and Pplat can be visualized and measured.
1st waveform: Ppeak − Pplat = 5 cmH$_2$O
2nd waveform: Ppeak − Pplat = 10 cmH$_2$O
Clinical Notes: An increased Ppeak while Plat remains the same is indicative of an increased Raw. The reverse situation, a decreased Ppeak while Pplat remains the same, is indicative of a decreased Raw (e.g., a positive bronchodilator response).

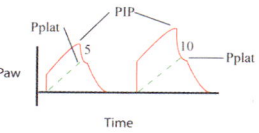

Volume-Time
The time for volume emptying is prolonged with increased Raw

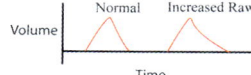

Flow-Time

A: normal
B: ↑ Raw (expiratory):
1) Peak expiratory flow is decreased
2) Expiratory flow is decreased (flatter slope)
3) Time of expiration is prolonged

Clinical Notes: Bronchodilator response is determined by the degree to which the increased Raw waveform returns to a normal shape. Inspiratory Raw is generally not well depicted on a flow-time scalar because ventilator-driving force is usually sufficient to overcome it.

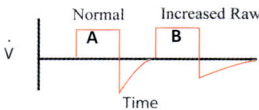

Pressure-Volume (ventilator breath)

The dashed line depicts a normal loop. The solid line depicts increased Raw. The movement of the upward inspiratory slope to the right is indicative of inspiratory resistance. The movement of the downward expiratory slope to the left is indicative of expiratory resistance.

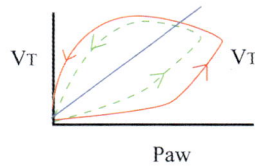

Pressure-Volume (spontaneous breath)

The inspiratory area (A) to the left of the vertical baseline will increase with increased inspiratory Raw. The expiratory area (B) to the right of the vertical baseline will increase with an increase in expiratory Raw.

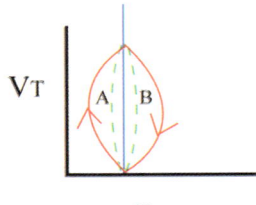

Flow-Volume

The dashed line depicts a normal loop. The solid line depicts increased Raw:

1. Decreased peak expiratory flow
2. Concave mid-expiratory flow curve (theoretically due to resistance in medium and small airways. No concavity suggests the resistance is in the large upper airways).
3. V_T may be reduced in some instances

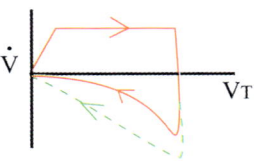

Clinical Notes: Bronchodilator response is determined by the degree to which the increased Raw waveform returns to a normal shape. Inspiratory Raw is generally not well depicted on a flow-volume loop because ventilator-driving force is usually sufficient to overcome it.

Compliance Changes
Possible Causes

Decreased	Increased
• ARDS • Atelectasis • Abdominal distention • CHF • Consolidation • Fibrosis • Hyperinflation • Pleural effusion • Right mainstem intubation • Tension pneumothorax	• Emphysema • Surfactant therapy

> Address the underlying issue when possible. Often compliance cannot be directly addressed. Consider tools to support the pathophysiology.

Pressure-Time

Using an inspiratory pause (hold), the difference between Ppeak and Pplat can be visualized and measured.

A: Ppeak – Pplat = 5 cmH$_2$O
B: Ppeak – Pplat = 5 cmH$_2$O

Clinical Notes:

If Ppeak and Pplat ↑ along with the Raw (Ppeak-Pplat), this is indicative of ↓ C and ↑ Raw.

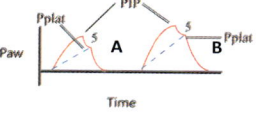

See airway resistance changes, previous section. Pressure curves remain unchanged in PV. An ↑ Ppeak plus a similar ↑ in Pplat is indicative of ↓ compliance.

The reverse situation, a ↓ Ppeak plus a similar ↓ in Pplat is indicative of an ↑ compliance.

Pressure-Volume

Decreasing compliance: the slope of the imaginary line through the center of the loop moves towards the pressure axis

Increasing compliance: the slope of the imaginary line through the center of the loop moves towards the volume axis.

Clinical Note: Depending on the parameters and scaling, normal compliance curves are conventionally displayed as having a 45° slope

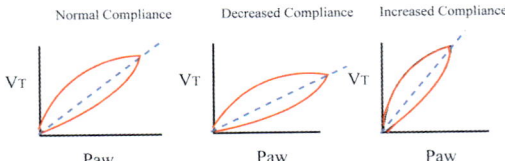

Excessive (Active) Exhalation

Possible Causes
- Patient is exhaling below functional residual capacity due to:
  - Air-trapping (excessive exhalation occurs periodically in an attempt to relieve the trapped volume).
  - Pain
  - Positional change

Note a consistent, regular pattern of excessive exhalation may indicate an equipment calibration problem.

Descriptions:

Volume-Time
Volume curve dips below zero baseline

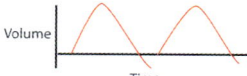

Pressure-Volume
Expiration curve continues below the zero volume point.

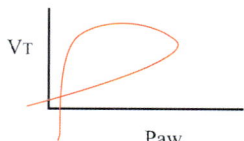

Flow-Volume
Expiration curve continues to the left of the zero volume point.

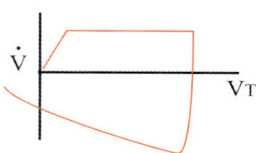

Graphics   5-43

Partial Obstruction

Possible Causes
- Indwelling suction catheter left partially in ET tube
- Flap of tissue, Mucous plug
- Water/secretions in airways/circuit

Flow-Time
The obstruction is moved by flow moving in and out of the airways/circuit resulting in fluctuating flow.

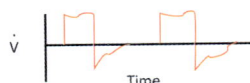

Pressure-Volume
The obstruction is moved by the flow moving in and out of the airways/circuit, resulting in fluctuating pressure.

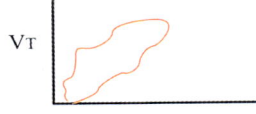

Flow-Volume
The obstruction is moved by the flow moving in and out of the airways/circuit, resulting in fluctuating flow. It will have a "saw tooth" appearance if the obstruction is secretions or water.

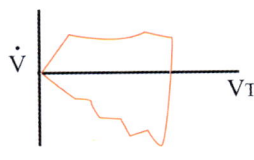

Overdistension

> The pressure-volume loop is typically used for identifying lower and higher inflection points (see page 7-26). Note that a specific ventilator tool is required to be accurate.
>
> When over-distension is suspected (especially if hemodynamic effects, such as hypotension), analyze VT or PIP. If appropriate, consider decreasing PEEP.

Possible Causes
- Excessive tidal volume (in volume modes)
- Excessive inspiratory pressure (in pressure modes)
- Excessive PEEP (beyond optimal)

Pressure-Volume
Increasing inspiratory pressure results in smaller-than-expected tidal volume increases. This can be seen as a "beaking" at end-inspiration (see arrow) Increasing volume increases pressure for a very little or no increase VT causing a "beaking" at end inspiration. Note that beaking may also occur with patient-ventilator asynchrony.

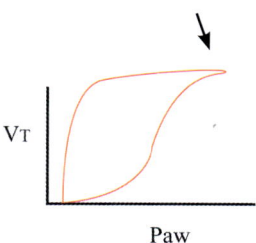

Leaks

Possible Causes

Expiratory	Inspiratory
• Air leak through chest tube • BP fistula • ET tube cuff leak • NG tube in trachea	• Loose connections • Ventilator malfunction • Faulty flow sensor

Clinical Note: Leaks are generally expiratory. Set volumes will not be reached if the leak is inspiratory. A leak in the circuit between the ventilator and flow transducer would result in a smaller volume (both I and E); pressure and flow are then set by the ventilator.

Pressure-Time
Ppeak will be ↓ (especially volume ventilation) due to ↓ returned volume and/or an inspiratory leak.

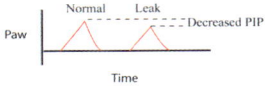

Volume-Time
Set volume is not reached with an inspiratory leak. The returned volume does not return to baseline with an expiratory leak.

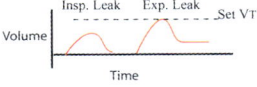

Flow-Time
Peak expiratory flow is ↓ due to ↓ returned volume.

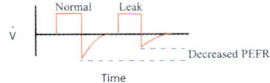

Pressure-Volume
Volume does not return to zero baseline, resulting in an incomplete loop. The dashed line depicts a loop without a leak.

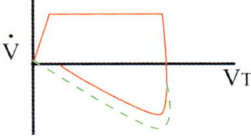

Flow-Volume
Volume does not return to zero baseline, resulting in an incomplete loop. The dashed line depicts a loop without a leak.

Rate Asynchrony

Possible Causes
- Neurological injury
- Patient air-hunger

Pressure-Time
Erratic inspiratory and/or expiratory phases indicate inspiratory and/or expiratory efforts to inhale or exhale.

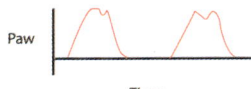

Flow-Time
Erratic inspiratory and/or expiratory phases indicate inspiratory and/or expiratory efforts to inhale or exhale.

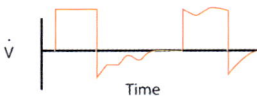

Pressure-Volume
Erratic inspiratory and/or expiratory phases indicate inspiratory and/or expiratory efforts to inhale or exhale.

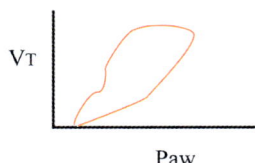

Flow-Volume
Erratic inspiratory and/or expiratory phases indicate inspiratory and/or expiratory efforts to inhale or exhale.

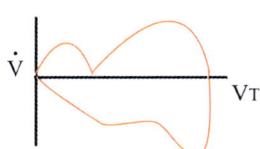

Flow Asynchrony (Flow Starvation)

Pressure-Time
The inspiratory limb is scooped with a negative pressure deflection due to the patient's attempt to pull more flow. The expiratory curve is unaffected by flow starvation.

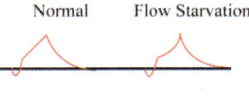

Adjusting Peak Flow:
In volume modes the rate of rise in pressure (upward slope) is determined in part by the peak flow setting. An inadequate flow presents as a slow and often scooped rise to peak pressure. A high flow will present as a very fast rise to peak pressure (similar to pressure modes).

Pressure-Volume
The inspiratory limb is concave with a negative pressure deflection due to the patient's attempt to pull more flow. The expiratory curve will be unaffected by flow starvation

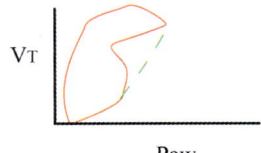

Trigger Asynchrony
(due to inappropriate trigger/sensitivity)

Pressure-Time
Negative inspiratory pressure is applied by the patient, however it is not enough to trigger a machine breath.

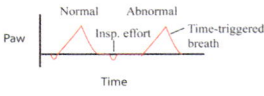

Flow-Time
As the patient attempts to trigger the ventilator, the flow turns slightly positive then negative due to a futile effort.

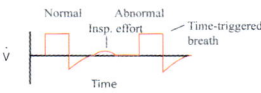

Pressure-Volume
Normal – the negative deflection is minimal.
Abnormal – the negative deflection is greater. The greater the negative deflection, the greater the effort to trigger.

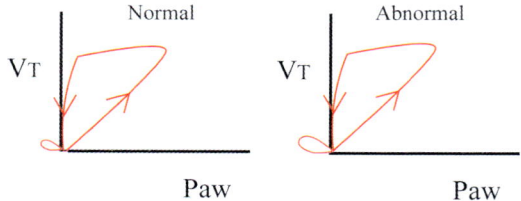

Trigger Asynchrony
(due to auto-PEEP)

Pressure-Time
Normal – the negative deflection is minimal.
Abnormal – the negative deflection is greater. The greater the negative deflection, the greater the effort to trigger.
Note that this graphic can't be differentiated in appearance from asynchrony due to an inappropriate trigger.

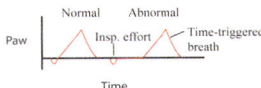

Flow-Time
As the patient attempts to trigger the ventilator, the expiratory flow curve turns slightly positive, then negative. This inspiratory effort does not result in triggering the ventilator.
Note the inspiratory effort below baseline (compare to the flow-time scalar on previous page)

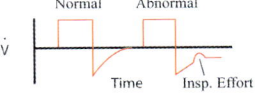

Select Other Uses for Graphics

Pressure-Time Scalars

Determining ventilator breath type (volume modes)
A negative pressure deflection just prior to inspiration indicates an assisted breath

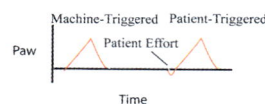

Assessing Plateau Pressure
In volume modes, an inspiratory pause will cause the pressure to plateau*

In pressure modes, PIP = Pplat*

*Note that flow needs to be absent at end-inspiration (so if the patient is making efforts, seen as an inconsistent plateau, the Pplat measurement is likely to be less accurate)

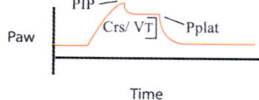

Setting rise-to-pressure time in pressure modes (controlled or supported)

The faster the flow, the quicker set pressure is reached in the I phase.

This is used in conjunction with the flow-time scalar (see next section). A rise-to-pressure time too fast could cause a spike or "ringing" in the airways and cause the patient to become asynchronous.

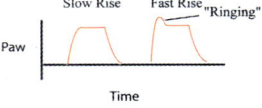

Switching cycling criteria and optimizing inspiratory phase in pressure support

Ventilators have specific flow-cycling criteria for pressure-supported breaths. Some ventilators have backup pressure and time-cycling features that can be adjusted. In the example shown, the first breath is pressure-cycled. Note the pressure spike at the end of inspiration, indicating that the flow-cycling parameter (e.g., 25%) is too low and that the patient is attempting to exhale. Adjusting the expiratory sensitivity or the time-cycling parameter, the clinician can limit the inspiratory phase, which may improve patient comfort.

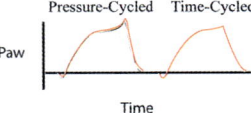

Flow-Time Scalars

Verifying waveform shapes
If flow waveform can be set, the flow-time scalar quickly identifies which. Note: decelerating flow is preferred clinically for a majority of patients.

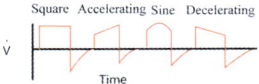

Setting inspiratory time (pressure modes)
When lengthening or shortening the inspiratory time, the flow-time scalar should be used to see if there is more flow available for additional volume delivery. Once the $\dot{V}I$ has reached zero (baseline), there will no further appreciable volume delivery gain.

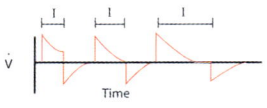

Setting rise-to-pressure time in pressure modes
The faster the flow, the quicker set pressure is reached in the inspiratory phase. Use this in combination with the pressure-time scalar (see previous page)

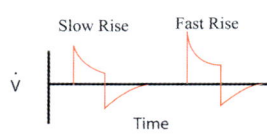

Pressure-Volume Loop

Assessing inspiratory effort
The clockwise loops below the baseline pressure depict patient inspiratory effort in assist ventilation.
- A (red): increased (inappropriate) trigger effort
- B (green): minimum (appropriate) trigger effort

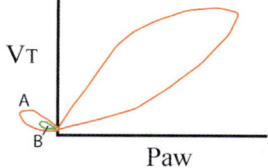

6 Equations

Acid-Base 6-2
Oxygenation 6-4
Ventilation 6-12
Ventilator Calculations
  General 6-16
  Weaning 6-17
  Mechanics 6-19
Hemodynamic Monitoring 6-23
Patient Calculations 6-29
  IBW and PBW 6-29
  Gas Duration 6-30

Equations

Acid-Base

Equation	Explanation	Clinical Application
Anion Gap	AG: the difference between measured cations (+) and anions (−) (the unmeasured ions)	Indicates whether a metabolic acidosis is due to an increase of acid (rather than a decrease of base)
$AG = Na^+ - (Cl^- + HCO_3^-)$ (United States)	Normal: 12 (± 4) mEq/L	↑ AG = ↑ unmeasured anions (acid): ↑ **acid production:** lactate (hypoxia) ketones (diabetes) ↑**acid addition:** poisons (methanol, salicylates) ↓ **acid excretion:** renal failure ↓ AG = ↓ unmeasured anions: albumin
$AG = (Na^+ + K^+) - (Cl^- + HCO_3^-)$ (International adds K+)	Normal: 16 (± 4) mEq/L	
Base Excess (BE)	To calculate base excess	May be used to help confirm validity of results
$BE = \dfrac{\Delta PaCO_2 + \Delta pH \times 100}{2}$	$\Delta PaCO_2$: change from normal (40) ΔpH: change from normal (7.40)	Accurate only in ranges of: $PaCO_2$: 30-50, pH 7.30-7.50

Equation	Explanation	Clinical Application
Henderson-Hasselbach $$pH = 6.1 + \log\left[\frac{HCO_3^-}{0.03 \times PCO_2}\right]$$	6.1: a dissociation constant HCO_3^-: bicarb level from ABG 0.03: the CO_2 solubility constant PCO_2: the partial pressure of CO_2	Calculation of pH or $PaCO_2$
Rule of 8s (HCO_3^- Estimation) | pH is: | multiply PaCO2 by: | |---|---| | 7.6 | 8/8 | | 7.5 | 6/8 | | 7.4 | 5/8 | | 7.3 | 4/8 | | 7.2 | 3/8 |	Example: pH: 7.4 PaCO2: 40 mmHg Multiply PaCO2 by 5/8 Estimated HCO_3^-: 25 mEq/L	When given the pH and $PaCO_2$, this estimates HCO_3^-. Use especially for verifying if an ABG is valid (see *Oakes' ABG Pocket Guide*)
Winters' Formula ($PaCO_2$ Estimation) $PaCO_2$ predicted $= 1.54 \times HCO_3^- + 8.36\ (\pm1)$	**Interpretation:** If actual $PaCO_2$ is greater than predicted, there is a mixed acidosis If actual $PaCO_2$ is less than predicted, there is a respiratory alkalosis	Measures respiratory compensation for metabolic acidosis

Equations

Equations

Equation	Explanation	Clinical Application
Oxygenation		
A-a O_2 Gradient $P(A-a)O_2$ $(A-a)DO_2$ = $P_AO_2 - P_aO_2$ **Estimate** Expected $P_AO_2 = 500 \times FiO_2$	Normal: 10 - 25 mmHg (air) = 30 - 50 mmHg (100% O_2) P_AO_2: Alveolar Air Equation (see below) P_aO_2: from ABG FiO_2: decimal form of O_2 Increases with age: Expected A-a gradient = (Age + 10) / 4	Assists in determining between a shunt and V/Q mismatch **Use when assessing hypoxia** (especially if unexplained or more severe than clinically expected) Increased Shunt, V/Q mismatch, alveolar hypoventilation, or ↓ diffusion
Alveolar Air Equation P_AO_2 = $([Pb - PH_2O] \times FiO_2) - PaCO_2/RQ$	Normal on RA = 100 mmHg on FiO_2 1.0 = 663 mmHg Pb: barometric pressure (mmHg) (sea level = 760) PH_2O: water vapor pressure (normal = 47) FiO_2: decimal form of O_2 $PaCO_2$: from ABG RQ: Respiratory Quotient (normal = 0.8)	The partial pressure of oxygen in the alveoli. This is an important value in determining how much oxygen is getting from the alveoli (P_AO_2) to arterial blood (P_aO_2). Assuming normal RQ, you can make this quicker by multiplying by an RQ of 1.25 instead of dividing by 0.8. Used in several equations: P(A-a)O_2 gradient, a/A ratio, and percentage shunt

Equation	Explanation	Clinical Application
Arterial/Alveolar O_2 Tension a/A Ratio $= PaO_2 / P_AO_2$	Normal: 0.8 - 0.9 at any FiO_2 (elderly may be lower, ~0.75) Index of gas exchange function or efficiency of the lungs	More stable than A-a gradient: A-a gradient changes with FiO_2, a/A remains relatively stable with FiO_2 changes. $PaCO_2$ or V/Q changes can alter <0.6 = shunt, V/Q mismatch, or diffusion defect; < 0.35 indicative of weaning failure <0.15 = refractory hypoxemia
Arterial-Venous O_2 Content Difference $C(a-\bar{v})O_2$ $= CaO_2 - C\bar{v}O_2$	Normal $C(a-\bar{v})O_2 = (20-15) = \sim 5$ vol% Difference between <u>arterial</u> and <u>mixed venous</u> O_2 contents. CaO_2: Arterial O_2 Content 20 vol% $C\bar{v}O_2$: Mixed Venous O_2 Content Normal = 15 vol%	Represents O_2 consumption by tissues, and an estimate of cardiac output **Increased** Decreased cardiac output Increased O_2 consumption (fever, etc.) **Decreased** Increased cardiac output Paralytics Peripheral shunting (sepsis, trauma)

Equation	Explanation	Clinical Application
FiO$_2$ Estimation Desired FiO$_2$ = $\dfrac{\text{Desired PaO}_2 \times \text{Known FiO}_2}{\text{Known PaO}_2}$	Desired FiO$_2$: "new" FiO$_2$ to set Desired PaO$_2$: goal PaO$_2$ Known FiO$_2$: current FiO$_2$ Known PaO$_2$: current PaO$_2$	Used to estimate the FiO$_2$ needed to achieve a target PaO$_2$. This is an estimate with some basic assumptions (for example, with a V/Q mismatch, increasing FiO$_2$ may not adequately raise PaO$_2$)
Oxygen Consumption (Demand) $\dot{V}O_2$ = CO × C(a-$\bar{v}$)O$_2$ × 10	CO: Cardiac Output C(a-$\bar{v}$)O$_2$: CaO$_2$ - C$\bar{v}$O$_2$ Normal: 200-250 mL/min $\dot{V}O_2$I **(Oxygen Consumption Index)** can be calculated by replacing CO with CI (Cardiac Index). This takes into account body size. Normal = 110-165 mL/min/m^2	Volume of oxygen consumed by the body tissues per minute. Indication of metabolic level and cardiac output **Increased** Increased metabolism Increased cardiac output **Decreased** Decreased metabolism Decreased cardiac output

Equations

Equation	Explanation	Clinical Application
Oxygen Content CaO_2 $C\bar{v}O_2$ CcO_2 (see each, below)	1.34: constant representing the amount of oxygen bound per gram of hemoglobin. Values from 1.34 - 1.39 are considered acceptable (references vary) Hgb: Hemoglobin 0.0031: constant representing the amount of oxygen dissolved in plasma	Oxygen Content represents the amount of oxygen bound to hemoglobin (the majority) + the amount of blood dissolved in plasma (minimal)
(Arterial Oxygen Content) $CaO_2 =$ $(Hgb \times 1.34 \times SaO_2) + (PaO_2 \times 0.003)$	Normal: 15-24 mL/dL (vol%) SaO_2: calculated in ABG PaO_2: from ABG	Useful in determining how much oxygen is actually in blood. Unlike PaO_2 or SaO_2, incorporates hemoglobin. Total amount of oxygen in arterial blood
(Mixed Venous Oxygen Content) $C\bar{v}O_2 =$ $(Hgb \times 1.34 \times S\bar{v}O_2) + (P\bar{v}O_2 \times 0.003)$	Normal: 12-15 mL/dL (vol%) $S\bar{v}O_2$: calculated in mixed venous blood gas $P\bar{v}O_2$: from mixed venous blood gas (PA catheter)	Total amount of oxygen in mixed venous blood
(Pulmonary Capillary Oxygen Content) $CcO_2 =$ $(Hgb \times 1.34 \times ScO_2) + (PAO_2 \times 0.003)$	ScO_2 is usually assumed to be 100% (so can be left out) PcO_2: PAO_2 for clinical purposes	Total amount of oxygen in capillary blood (before anatomical shunts)

Equations

Equation	Explanation	Clinical Application
Oxygen Delivery (Supply) $\dot{D}O_2$ $= CO \times CaO_2 \times 10$	Normal: 750-1000 mL/min CO: Cardiac Output CaO_2: O_2 Content (see equation) 10: conversion factor to mL/min $\dot{D}O_2i$ (**O_2 Delivery Index**) can be calculated by dividing $\dot{D}O_2$ by BSA (accounts for body size) Normal is 500-600 mL/min/m²	The amount of oxygen is transported from the lungs to the circulation **Increased:** Hyperoxia, FiO_2, ECMO **Decreased:** Cardiac Output decreases (cardiac, hypovolemia, etc.), respiratory disorder (V/Q mismatch, diffusion issue, hypoventilation)
O_2 Extraction Ratio O_2ER $= \dfrac{O_2 \text{ demand } (\dot{V}O_2)}{O_2 \text{ supply } (\dot{D}O_2)}$ $= \dfrac{C(a-\overline{v})O_2}{CaO_2}$	Normal: ~25 % ($\dot{V}O_2$: ~250 mL/min, $\dot{D}O_2$: ~1 L/min) Ratio of the body's oxygen consumption ($\dot{V}O_2$) to systemic oxygen delivery ($\dot{D}O_2$) Actual O_2ER also varies by organ	Indicator of the adequacy of systemic oxygen delivery. Normal resting $\dot{D}O_2$ is usually more than adequate to meet $\dot{V}O_2$ (ensuring aerobic metabolism). As demand ($\dot{V}O_2$) increases or delivery ($\dot{D}O_2$) decreases, O_2ER increases to maintain aerobic metabolism until ~70% (max O_2ER). After this, anaerobic metabolism/tissue hypoxia is likely **Increased:** Decreased oxygen delivery or increased oxygen consumption **Decreased:** Increased oxygen delivery or decreased oxygen consumption

Equation	Explanation	Clinical Application
Oxygen Index (Oxygenation Index) OI $$= \frac{FiO_2 \times 100 \times \overline{Paw}}{PaO_2}$$	Normal = no defined normal, but lower is better (OI is close to 0 if all parameters are physiologic/normal) FiO_2: use decimal form $\overline{Paw}$: Mean Airway Pressure* PaO_2: from ABG A noninvasive form of OI, Oxygen Saturation Index (OSI), substitutes SpO_2 for PaO_2.	Helpful in assessing severity of hypoxia. Unlike P/f ratio, takes mean airway pressure into account (PEEP, etc.) Used clinically to help guide therapies such as nitric oxide, surfactant and ECMO • Signs of refractory hypoxemia at around 10-15 • Higher OI (25 or higher) may indicate severe hypoxemic respiratory failure
Oxygen Reserve $= \dot{D}O_2 - \dot{V}O_2$	Normal: 750 mL/min $= CO \times C\overline{v}O_2 \times 10$	Venous O_2 supply: O_2 supply minus O_2 demand
Oxygen Saturation (mixed venous) $S\overline{v}O_2$ $= SaO_2 - \dot{V}O_2/\dot{D}O_2$	Normal: 75 % (60-80 %)	Percent of hemoglobin saturated with oxygen (in mixed venous blood)

*The abbreviation for mean airway pressure, $\overline{Paw}$ can also be written as MAP, but because that is also used to refer to mean arterial pressure, this book uses $\overline{Paw}$ to refer to mean airway pressure, MAP to mean mean arterial pressure

Equation	Explanation	Clinical Application
Oxygen Saturation SaO_2 $= HbO_2 / \text{Total Hb} \times 100$	Normal: 95-100% HbO_2: Oxyhemoglobin Content	Percentage of hemoglobin that is occupied (usually by oxygen) May be falsely elevated by abnormal hemoglobins (carbon monoxide, etc.)
P/F Ratio (PaO_2/FiO_2 ratio, Horowitz Index) $= PaO_2 / FiO_2$	Normal: 400-500 mmHg PaO_2: from ABG FiO_2: in decimal format	This is a basic estimate of the A-a gradient, used at bedside because it is a simple calculation. Used with other criteria for determining ARDS severity (Berlin definition): | P/F Ratio	Severity
---	---
200-300	Mild
100-200	Moderate
< 100	Severe	 Both mortality and ventilator days increase as the P/F ratio drops (especially below 200)

Equation	Explanation	Clinical Application
Predicted PaO2 in Adults (based on age) Predicted PaO$_2$ = 109 - 0.4 (Age in Years)	Age | Expected PaO$_2$ 30 | 97 40 | 93 50 | 89 60 | 85 70 | 81 80 | 77	Use this as a rough estimate (there are other equations that will produce slightly different numbers, but these are all estimates) PaO$_2$ decreases as people age due to changes in lung mechanics (such as a decreasing $\dot{V}/\dot{Q}$)
Respiratory Index RI = $P(A-a)O_2 / PaO_2$	Normal: < 1.0	Estimation of oxygenation 1.0 - 5.0 = V/Q mismatch > 5.0 = refractory hypoxemia due to physiological shunt
Respiratory Quotient (Exchange ratio) (RQ, RE) RQ = $\dot{V}CO_2 / \dot{V}O_2$	Normal: 200 / 250 = 0.8 While $\dot{V}CO_2$ and $\dot{V}O_2$ are in ml/min, the actual quotient has no unit RQ = ratio of CO_2 produced to O_2 consumed (internal respiration) RE = the amount of O_2/CO_2 exchange in the lungs per minute (external respiration) RE = RQ in steady state condition	RQ is an indicator of the balance between O_2 being used and CO_2 being produced. Indirect calorimetry is used to collect the information needed

Equation	Explanation	Clinical Application
Ventilation		
Alveolar (Minute) Ventilation $\dot{V}_A$ $= \dot{V}_E - \dot{V}_D$	Normal: 4-6 L/min $\dot{V}_E$: Minute ventilation $\dot{V}_D$: Dead space ventilation As the equation shows, dead space ventilation is subtracted from minute ventilation, leaving alveolar ventilation	The volume of inspired air reaching the alveoli **per minute** By definition $\dot{V}_A < \dot{V}_E$ (due to dead space)
Alveolar Volume V_A $= \dot{V}_A / f$	$\dot{V}_A$: Alveolar ventilation f: Frequency (respiratory rate)	The volume of inspired air reaching the alveoli **per breath**
Dead Space Ventilation $\dot{V}_D$ $= \dot{V}_E - \dot{V}_A$	Normal: 1/3 $\dot{V}_E$ $\dot{V}_E$: Minute ventilation $\dot{V}_A$: Alveolar ventilation	The volume of wasted air (not participating in gas exchange) per minute

Equation	Explanation	Clinical Application
Dead Space Volume V_D $= V_T - V_A$ See nomogram, next page	Normal: 1/3 V_T Anatomical: 1 mL/lb IBW = 0.5 mL/lb w/ art. airway Mechanical: ~ 10 mL/inch of tubing	The volume of wasted air (not participating in gas exchange) per breath (V > Q) Increased: ↓ CO, pulmonary vasoconstriction, pulmonary embolus
Dead Space / V_T Volume Ratio V_D/V_T	Normal: 0.33 (150 V_D /450 V_T)	Used to measure the portion of V_T not participating in gas exchange (wasted ventilation) $V_D/V_T > 0.5$ is indicative of respiratory failure
Physiological V_D/V_T Ratio (Bohr Equation): $\dfrac{V_{Dphys}}{V_T} = \dfrac{P_aCO_2 - P_{\bar{E}}CO_2}{P_aCO_2}$	$P_{\bar{E}}CO_2$: mixed expired Estimate: $V_{Dphys} / V_T =$ ($\dot{V}_E$ actual / $\dot{V}_E$ predicted) x (P_aCO_2 actual / 40) x 0.33	*Technically, P_aCO_2 would best reflect deadspace but can't be measured reliably (and often varies from one alveolus to the next). Clinically, P_aCO_2 is used as a rough estimation of the impact of dead space. Many lung diseases (atelectasis, pneumonia, pulmonary edema, emboli, etc.) can exhibit changes in V_D (i.e., V_{Dalv}) without corresponding changes in P_aCO_2*
Anatomical V_D/V_T Ratio: $\dfrac{V_{Danat}}{V_T} = \dfrac{PetCO_2 - P_{\bar{E}}CO_2}{PetCO_2}$	Pet: end tidal	

Nomogram to estimate minute ventilation required to maintain a given PaCO2 when VD/VT is known:

To obtain the required minute ventilation to achieve a given PaCO2, the minute ventilation is plotted against the PaCO2 (measured simultaneously) and the VD/VT ratio is read on the isopleth that corresponds to the intersection. The isopleth is then followed to the desired PaCO2 and the corresponding minute ventilation read off the vertical axis.

For example: A patient with a $\dot{V}_E$ of 5L and a PaCO2 of 60 mmHgs has an estimated VD/VT ratio of 0.40. To achieve a desired PaCO2 of 40 mmHg, follow the 0.40 isopleth up to correspond to the PaCO2 of 40 on the horizontal axis. Then read the appropriate minute ventilation of about 8 L/min off the vertical axis.

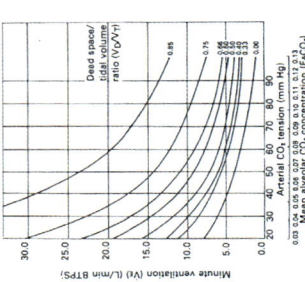

Equation	Explanation	Clinical Application
Minute Ventilation (Minute Volume) $\dot{V}_E$ = $V_T \times f$	Normal: 5 - 7 L/min V_T: Tidal Volume f: Frequency (Respiratory Rate)	Total amount of gas moved into (inhaled minute ventilation) or out of (exhaled minute ventilation) the lungs per minute With modes that allow for calculate set breaths be sure to calculate set breaths (f and average V_T) and spontaneous breaths (f and average V_T)

6-14 Equations

Equation	Explanation	Clinical Application
Ventilation/Perfusion Ratio $\dot{V}/\dot{Q}$ Ratio $$\dot{V}_A/\dot{Q}c = \frac{(C\bar{v}CO_2 - CaCO_2) \times 8.63}{PaCO_2}$$	Normal: $\frac{4L/min}{5L/min} = 0.8$ Ratio of minute alveolar ventilation to minute capillary blood flow Represents external respiration	Ratio changes represent the degree and type of respiratory imbalances ↓ Ratio (↓V/Q) = atelectasis, COPD, pneumonia, pneumothorax, N-M disorders, etc. ↑ Ratio (V/↓Q) = shock, pulmonary emboli, cor pulmonale, PPV

Equation	Explanation	Clinical Application
Ventilator Calculations		
Equation of Motion Pvent= $(\dot{V} \times R) + (V \times E) + PEEP$	Pvent = Peak pressure $\dot{V}$ = Flow R = Resistance V = Volume E = Elastance (inverse of compliance)	While typically not used clinically, referring to and understanding this equation is a foundation to understanding ventilators
Ventilator Flow $\dot{V} =$ $\dot{V}_E \times RFF$	RFF = Ratio Flow Factor (I + E from I:E ratio)	Used to calculate appropriate flow for delivering a given tidal volume (Vt) in a given inspiratory time (Ti)
Ventilator Rate Determination New Rate = $\dfrac{\text{Current Rate} \times \text{Known PaCO}_2}{\text{Desired PaCO}_2}$	Rate can be exchanged with $\dot{V}_E$ New $\dot{V}_E =$ $\dfrac{\text{Current } \dot{V}_E \times \text{Known PaCO}_2}{\text{Desired PaCO}_2}$	Assumes a steady metabolic rate with no spontaneous breaths If assist-control mode, be sure to calculate based on total (set + patient-triggered) rate, not set rate

Equation	Explanation	Clinical Application
Weaning Calculations		
CORE Index = $C_{dyn} \times (PI_{max}/P0.1) \times (PaO_2/PAO_2)/f$	C = Compliance (Cdyn) O = Oxygenation (PaO_2/PAO_2) R = Rate (f) E = Effort ($PI_{max}/P0.1$)	8 or below may indicate weaning failure
CROP Index = $\dfrac{C_{dyn} \times (PaO_2/PAO_2) \times PI_{max}}{Rate}$	C = Compliance (Cdyn) R = Rate (f) O = Oxygenation (PaO_2/PAO_2) P = Pressure (PI_{max})	< 13 may indicate weaning failure
Integrative Weaning Index IWI = $(C_{stat} \times SaO_2) / (f/V_T)$		< 25 may indicate weaning failure

Equation	Explanation	Clinical Application
Rapid Shallow Breathing Index RSBI $= f / V_T$	Measure f and V_T (in liters) while receiving no or minimal vent support (usually CPAP) Some clinicians prefer to use a spirometer attached to the artificial airway	A higher RSBI suggests readiness to extubate <100-105 breaths/min/L suggests weaning success (on a T-Piece) <75 breaths/min/L is the threshold suggested in some evidence for patients on low amounts of PSV or on CPAP See clinical notes on RSBI (pg 11-19)
Simplified Weaning Index SWI= $f(\text{mech}) \times (\text{PIP-PEEP} / \text{PIMax}) \times (\text{PaCO}_2 / 40)$	Simplified version of the more complex "weaning index"	Acceptable = under 9 Failure = higher than 11

Equation	Explanation	Clinical Application
Mechanics		
Airway Resistance Raw $= \text{PIP} - \text{Pplat} / \dot{V}_I$	Normal: 0.5 - 2.5 cmH$_2$O/L/sec @ a flow of 0.5 L/sec (30 L/min) with ET tube (properly sized) = 4 - 8 cmH$_2$O/L/sec PIP: Peak Inspiratory Pressure Pplat: Plateau Pressure $\dot{V}_I$: Inspiratory Flow in L/sec ↑PIP + ↑Pplat (P$_{TA}$ constant) = ↓Cstat ↑PIP + same Pplat (↑P$_{TA}$) = ↑Raw ↓PIP + ↓Pplat (P$_{TA}$ constant) = ↑Cstat ↓PIP + same Pplat (↓P$_{TA}$) = ↓Raw	Represents frictional resistance of airflow (80%) and tissue motion (20%) **Increased airflow resistance**: trachea (normal resistance from turbulent airflow), airway collapse (tracheomalacia, etc.), edema, bronchospasm, secretions, artificial airway (ET tube) **Increased tissue resistance**: pulmonary edema, fibrosis, pneumonia Small changes in radius will increase airway resistance dramatically Technically there exists both inspiratory (RI) and expiratory resistance (RE). They approximate each other normally, but may vary with lung disease. This equation (since it uses inspiratory flow) measures inspiratory airway resistance.

Equation	Explanation	Clinical Application
Compliance	Normal: 70 - 100 mL/cmH$_2$O	Represents the ease of distention of the lungs and thorax
C	Total compliance can be referred to as Crs (respiratory system)	Includes elastic, functional, and tissue viscous resistance
$= \Delta V / \Delta P$	C$_{LT}$: lung + thorax	
	Compliances	Ideal = 100 mL/cmH$_2$O
C$_{LT}$ = C$_L$ + C$_{CW}$	C$_L$: lung compliance	
C$_L$ = ΔV / Palv - Ppl	C$_{CW}$: chest wall (thorax) compliance	Lungs and chest wall each = 200 mL/cmH$_2$O.
C$_{CW}$ = ΔV / Ppl - PB		
	Pressures	
See next pages for static/dynamic compliance	P$_B$ = barometric pressure	
	Ppl = pleural pressure	
	Palv = alveolar pressure	

Equation	Explanation	Clinical Application
Static Compliance C_{stat} $= V_T / P_{plat} - PEEP$	Normal: 70 - 100 mL/cmH$_2$O Pplat: inspiratory hold on ventilator until pressure stabilizes (1-4 seconds)	See also pg 4-13 Represents the combination of lung elasticity and chest wall recoil **Increased** ↑ lung elasticity or ↑ chest wall recoil. **Decreased** ↓ lung elasticity or ↓ chest wall recoil. Trending Cstat has greater value than interpreting a single value
Dynamic Compliance C_{dyn} $= V_T / PIP - PEEP$	Normal: 40 - 70 mL/cmH$_2$O	See also pg 4-13 Represents the combination of static lung compliance (Cstat) and airway resistance (Raw) Trending Cdyn has greater value than interpreting a single value

Equation	Explanation	Clinical Application
Driving Pressure ΔP = Pplat - PEEP	$\Delta P = V_T / C_{RS}$ (theoretical equation) Pplat: Plateau Pressure V_T: Tidal Volume C_{RS}: Respiratory System Compliance	May be a better measure of "functional" lung size (and is preferred by some in targeting safe V_T - versus using PBW or IBW) > 15 may increase mortality
Mean Airway Pressure $\overline{P}aw$, mPAW, MAP Constant Flow Volume Ventilation: = $0.5 \times (PIP-PEEP) \times (T_I/T_{tot}) + PEEP$	Average airway pressure (cmH2O) during several breathing cycles For pressure ventilation, use same equation but do not multiply by 0.5	Usually measured during mechanical ventilation, often used to monitor and indirectly manipulate oxygenation. PEEP is a major determinant If inspiratory and expiratory airway resistance are different (such as with lung disease), mean alveolar pressure may vary from mPAW

Equation	Explanation	Clinical Application
Time Constant TC TC = Raw × Cstat Note: TC generally refers to inspiratory TC. Expiratory TC may be much longer than inspiratory TC in COPD.	1TC = 63% 2TC = 87% 3TC = 95% 4TC = 98% 5TC = 99% %: % of V_T entering lungs within each TC period Normal TC = 0.2 sec Normal T_i = 3 - 4 TC = 3 or 4 × 0.2 sec = 0.6 – 0.8 sec	TC_{inspir} indicates alveolar filling time. ↑TC (> 0.2 sec) is usually indicative of ↑Raw (but may be ↑C). ↓TC (< 0.2 sec) is usually indicative of ↓C (but may be ↓Raw) TC_{expir} indicates alveolar emptying time Less than 3 TC_{expir} will generally result in air-trapping TC_{expir} may be approximated with a flow-volume loop
Perfusion/Hemodynamic Monitoring		
Cardiac Output CO or $\dot{Q}_T$ = SV × HR	Normal: 4-8 L/min (at rest) See Fick equation below and *Oakes' Hemodynamic Monitoring Pocket Guide* for more information. Cardiac Index (CI) can be calculated by dividing CO by BSA (takes into account body size)	Amount of blood ejected from heart per minute. Indicator of pump efficiency and a determinant of tissue perfusion

Equation	Explanation	Clinical Application
Fick Equation $\dot{V}O_2$ $= CO \times Ca\text{-}\bar{v}O_2$	See *Oakes' Hemodynamic Monitoring: A Bedside Reference Manual* for more info.	Method of measuring cardiac output. Fick estimate: $CO = 125 \times BSA / Ca\text{-}\bar{v}O_2$
Left Ventricular Stroke Work LVSW $= (MAP - PCWP) \times SV \times 0.0136$	Normal: 60–80 gm/m/beat MAP: Mean Arterial Pressure PCWP: Pulmonary Capillary Wedge Pressure (aka PAOP) SV: Stroke Volume To calculate the Index (LVSWI) substitute SV with SVI (takes body size into account)	Measure of pumping function of left ventricle = left ventricular contractility
Mean Arterial (Blood) Pressure (MAP, $\overline{BP}$) $= \dfrac{Systolic + 2(Diastolic)}{3}$	Normal: 93 mmHg (70–105) Systolic: top number in BP Diastolic: bottom number in BP	Average driving force of systemic circulation. A minimal MAP of about 60 is required to maintain sufficient perfusion to vital organs. Determined by cardiac output and total peripheral resistance.

Equation	Explanation	Clinical Application
Mean Pulmonary Artery Pressure $\overline{PAP}$, PAMP $$= \frac{PASP + 2(PADP)}{3}$$	Normal: 10-15 mmHg PASP: Pulmonary Artery Systolic Pressure PADP: Pulmonary Artery Diastolic Pressure	Average driving force of blood from the right heart to left heart (this is the pulmonary circulation)
Pulmonary Vascular Resistance PVR $$PVR = \frac{PAMP - PCWP}{CO} \times 80$$	Normal: 20-250 dynes•sec•cm^{-5} = 0.25-2.5 units (mmHg/L/min) PAMP: Pulmonary Artery Pressure Mean PCWP: Pulmonary Capillary Wedge Pressure CO: Cardiac Output To calculate the Index (PVRI) substitute CO with CI (takes body size into account)	Resistance to right ventricular ejection of blood into pulmonary vasculature Indicator of RV afterload

Equation	Explanation	Clinical Application
Pulse Pressure PP = BPsys - BPdia	Normal: 40 mmHg (20-80)	Difference between BP systolic and BP diastolic
Right Ventricular Stroke Work RVSW = (PAMP - CVP) x SV x 0.0136	Normal: 10-15 gm/m/beat PAMP: Pulmonary Artery Mean Pressure CVP: Central Venous Pressure SV: Stroke Volume To calculate the Index (RVSWI) divide RVSW by BSA (takes body size into account)	Measure of pumping function of right ventricle (RV contractility)

Equation	Explanation	Clinical Application
Shunt Equation $\dot{Q}_S/\dot{Q}_T$ **Clinical Equation (use if PaO$_2$ > 150)** $$= \frac{P(A-a)O_2 \times 0.003}{C(a-\bar{v})O_2 + P(A-a)O_2 \times 0.003}$$ **Classical Equation (use if PaO$_2$ < 150)** $$\frac{CcO_2 - CaO_2}{CcO_2 - CvO_2}$$ **Estimates** (ideal: FiO$_2$ 0.50 x 20 min before sampling/calculating) $= \frac{P(A-a)O_2}{20}$ $\dot{Q}_S/\dot{Q}_T$ = 5% per every 100 mmHg below expected	Normal: 2-5% (mostly from Thebesian veins) Ratio of shunted blood (Qs) to total cardiac output (QT) P(A-a)O$_2$: A-a O$_2$ Gradient C(a-$\bar{v}$)O$_2$: Arterial-Venous O$_2$ Content CcO$_2$: Pulmonary Capillary Oxygen Content CaO$_2$: Arterial Oxygen Content CvO$_2$: Mixed Venous Oxygen Content Estimate using PaO$_2$/FIO$_2$: > 300 = < 15% shunt 200 - 300 = 15 - 20% shunt < 200 = > 20% shunt C(a-$\bar{v}$)O$_2$ can be assumed if a mixed venous sample cannot be obtained: 4.5 - 5% if good CO and perfusion 3.5% in critically ill patients	A measure of right-to-left shunted blood (passes from right side of heart to left side of heart without being oxygenated, either for anatomical or physiological reasons) Indicator or efficiency of pulmonary system: < 10% = normal lungs 10-20% = minimal effect 20-30% = significant pulmonary disease > 30% = life-threatening This is a complicated calculation that requires a PA catheter to be more than an estimate. While the equation is uncommonly used, the concept is critical to bedside care.

Equation	Explanation	Clinical Application
Stroke Volume SV = CO/HR x 1000	Normal: 60-120 mL/beat CO: Cardiac Output HR: Heart Rate To calculate the Index (SVI) divide SV by BSA (takes body size into account)	Amount of blood ejected by either ventricle per contraction
Systemic Vascular Resistance SVR = $\dfrac{\text{MAP - CVP}}{\text{CO}}$ x 80	Normal: 800-1600 dynes•sec•cm^{-5} MAP: Mean Arterial Pressure CVP: Central Venous Pressure CO: Cardiac Output To calculate the Index (SVRI) substitute CO with CI (takes body size into account)	Resistance to LV ejection of blood into systemic circulation. Indicator of LV afterload. mmHg/L/min x 80 = dynes•sec•cm^{-5}

Equation	Explanation	Clinical Application
Patient Calculations		
Body Surface Area BSA $= (H^{0.725} \times W^{0.425}) \times 0.007184$	Average: 1.9 m² (males) 1.6 m² (females) H: Height in centimeters W: Weight in kilograms	When used with hemodynamic equations (usually then called an "index"), body size is at least partially accounted for (theoretically making the values more accurate)
Ideal Body Weight IBW (kg) IBW (female) kg = 45.5 + [0.9 × (Height in cm - 154)] IBW (male) kg = 50 + [0.9 × (Height in cm - 154)] **Estimate** (must convert to kg after. 1 kg = 2.2 lb) F: 100 + 5 lb per inch over 5 ft M: 106 + 6 lb per inch over 5 ft		IBW and PBW use calculations that are very similar. When used to calculate tidal volumes IBW underestimates the values (see pg 2-7) ARDSnet calculations are technically based upon PBW and some clinicians prefer using PBW for ventilator calculations. Using IBW will result in a slightly lower calculated VT (see pg 2-7 for VT calculations)
Predicted Body Weight PBW (kg) PBW (female) kg = 45.5 + [0.91 × (Height in cm - 152.4)] PBW (male) kg = 50 + [0.91 × (Height in cm - 152.4)]		

Equation	Explanation	Clinical Application
Gas Cylinder Duration Times Time (min) = $\dfrac{(\text{PSIG} - 500) \times \text{CF}}{\text{Flow (L/min)}}$	PSIG: Pressure from Cylinder 500: optional reserve (to ensure adequate supply, tank doesn't run dry) CF: conversion factor (L/psi)	**Oxygen Conversion Factors** D cyl: 0.16 (max PSIG: 2015) E cyl: 0.28 (max PSIG: 2015) H cyl: 3.14 (max PSIG: 2265) **Heliox Conversion Factors** E cyl: 0.23 (max PSIG: 2015) H cyl: 2.50 (max PSIG: 2265)
Duration of a Liquid System Amt of Gas (L) = $\dfrac{\text{Liquid Weight (lb)} \times 860}{2.5 \text{ lb/L}}$ Duration of Gas (min) = $\dfrac{\text{Amt of Gas (L)}}{\text{Flow (L/min)}}$	1 L liquid = 860 L gas Liquid Wt = Total Wt − Cylinder Wt	

7 Clinical Management

Airway Management
Bag-Valve-Mask 7-2
Airway Adjuncts 7-3
Endotracheal Tubes 7-4
   Intubation 7-5
Tracheostomy Tubes 7-8

Ventilation Management
Improving 7-15
Acute Respiratory Acidosis 7-16
Acute Respiratory Alkalosis 7-18
Metabolic Disorders 7-19
Permissive Hypercapnia 7-20

Oxygenation Management
Improving 7-21
Estimates 7-21
Strategies for Improving 7-22
PEEP 7-24

Airway Clearance Management
Suctioning 7-37
Other Methods 7-39

Humidity Management
Overview 7-42

Patient/Ventilator Synchrony
Artificial Airway 7-45
Auto-PEEP 7-45
Expiratory Valves 7-46
Humidifier 7-46
Trigger Sensitivity 7-47
Mode Asynchrony 7-49
Flow Asynchrony 7-50
Cycle Asynchrony 7-50

Airway Management
Bag-Valve-Mask (BVM) Ventilation

Variable	Considerations	
Rates	**General**	Adult: 10-12 breaths/min (every 5-6 sec) Pediatric: 20-30/min (every 2-3 sec)
	COPD **Raw ↑** **Hypovolemia**	6-8 breaths/min (every 7-10 sec) *minimizes Auto-PEEP*
	Adult CPR	No Airway: 30:2 ratio Airway: 10/min (every 6 sec) *allows for venous return*
Volumes	Estimated (deliver enough for visible chest rise):	
	Adult	Visible chest rise 500-600 mL (6-7 mL/kg) 1 L Adult Bag: 1/2 - 2/3 volume 2 L Adult Bag: 1/3 volume
	Infant/ Child	Visible Chest Rise Bag size should be < 450-500 mL
Gas Source	Usually connected to oxygen (commonly 15 L/min). Verify flow is from Oxygen outlet/tank, verify tubing is connected	
Personnel	1 Person: Ensure adequate airway position Use C:E technique to ensure mask seal Most effective with 2 Rescuers - 1 opens airway/seals mask, 2nd squeezes bag while both observe chest rise	
Risks	• Avoid high rates: higher rates may decrease venous return to the heart, decreasing coronary/cerebral perfusion • Avoid large volumes: risk of gastric insufflation (mask) or lung injury (mask or artificial airway)	
Inadequate Ventilation	• General deterioration (SpO$_2$, ETCO$_2$, HR, BP) • Decreased (or absent) breath sounds, chest rise	

Airway Adjuncts

Adjunct	Indications/Complications	Procedure
Nasopharyngeal Airway (NPA, Nasal Trumpet)	• Facilitates (nasotracheal) suctioning when required frequently (helps prevent trauma to the nares) • Assists in relieving upper airway obstruction in a conscious or unconscious patient (esp. tongue against posterior pharyngeal wall) Complications: Epistaxis, sinusitis	1. Determine correct size* (tip of nose to tragus of the ear) 2. Lubricate NPA (water soluble lubricant) 3. Inspect nares, use widest 4. Insert NPA with bevel towards septum, following the curvature of the nasal cavity floor, twisting gently to advance through the turbinates. If obstructed, try other naris. 5. If left in place, monitor skin integrity, switch nares every 8-12 hrs
Oropharyngeal Airway (OPA)	• Assists in relieving upper airway obstructions in an **unconscious** patient (often to facilitate bag-valve-mask ventilation) • Bite block with ET tube** Complications: gag/vomit	1. Note: patient must be unconscious/no gag reflex noted 2. Determine correct size* (corner of mouth to earlobe) 3. Insert with curve upward or lateral, then gently rotate curve to be towards the tongue 4. Should be used short-term, monitor skin integrity closely

Too small: will not prevent obstructing; Too large: may occlude the airway, cause gastric distension

** If used as a bite block, use very temporarily due to higher risk of skin breakdown than with commercial bite block designs

Management

Endotracheal Tubes (ET Tubes)

Types:
- Regular (with Murphy Eye), usually slightly curved, pliable
- Subglottic tubes (allow for suction above the cuff)
- Anti-aspiration designs (microcuff, silver-coated, etc.)
- Reinforced with metal coiling (if kinked, must replace)

Typical Sizing

	ET Tube I.D.(mm)	Avg Depth	Blade	Mask	Suction Catheter*(Fr)
Adult Male	6.5-9.5	21-23	3-4	4	8-14
Adult Female	6.0-8.5	19-21	3	4	8-12

* While suction catheter size should be determined by patient response, a starting point can be calculated using the formula: **[(ET Tube Size in mm) x 3] / 2, then choose closest even number (at or below)**

1 FR = 3 mm.

Modified Mallampati Scoring for Predicting a Difficult Airway

I	II	III	IV
Soft palate visible	Soft palate visible	Soft palate visible	Soft palate NOT visible
Uvula visible Pillars visible	Uvula visible	Base of uvula visible	Uvula NOT visible
Generally uncomplicated airway management		Potentially difficult airway management (including intubation)	

Management

Intubation

Equipment
Prepare and check all equipment
- Bag and valve mask ventilation (BVM)
  - connected/running on oxygen (12-15 L/min)
- Laryngoscope
  - check function of light/video
- Laryngoscope blades (Miller or MacIntosh)
- Endotracheal Tube (several sizes) with stylet
  - check cuff patency
  - use new endotracheal tube on each Intubation attempt
  - place stylet in endotracheal tube, if using
  - Lubricate the ET tube using water-soluble lubricant
- 10-cc Syringe
- Suction (rigid tonsillar suction connected and running)
- Waveform capnography running and ready
  - If unavailable, consider qualitative (e.g. Easy Cap) or Esophageal Detector Device (EDD)

Procedure
1. Ensure equipment is setup and checked
2. Position patient in sniffing position
3. Assess for difficult airway (see previous page)
4. Open mouth of patient (thumb-index-finger technique)
5. Insert laryngoscope blade, pulling upward and outward (keep wrist straight/rigid; do not pivot wrist)
6. Suction as needed
7. Insert the ET tube, watching specifically for indicator marks to go through the vocal cords
8. Inflate ET tube cuff with 10-cc syringe
9. Hold tube while removing laryngoscope and pulling stylet out
10. Attach BVM to tube
11. Verify tube placement (see checklist, next page)
12. Verify tube position (insertion distance from teeth should be around 19-21 cm female, 21-23 cm male)
13. Secure ET tube using commercial holder or tape

Confirmation of Tracheal Intubation Checklist:

Visualize Vocal Cords as Tube Passes Through	The best indicator of successful placement is visualization of tube going through vocal cords (preferably by 2 people)
Continuous Quantitative Waveform Capnography	Assumes adequate perfusion • This is the preferred method for verification (AHA) • Normal waveform/number should be present to confirm presence of CO_2
Qualitative Capnography (See next page)	Assumes adequate perfusion • The use of a device that changes color with CO_2 (yellow indicates CO_2 in most)
Esophageal Detector Device (See next page)	Less reliable than capnography but may be considered per (AHA) ACLS guidelines
Upper Airway Ultrasonography	Consider instead of capnography if inadequate perfusion (shock, cardiac arrest) • Enables visualization of upper airway structures to identify tube placement
Note Chest Rise	Should be bilateral, adequate rise *If R > L, suspect right mainstem intubation*
Vitals and Patient Color	Should be normal to ethnicity; pallor/cyanosis can be indicators of tube not in place
Auscultate over Chest Wall	Should be equal and bilateral breath sounds *If R > L suspect right mainstem intubation* *If both R + L ↓ suspect ET tube not in trachea*
Auscultate Epigastrium	No "breath sounds" in abdomen Some gurgling is normal
ET Tube	Note warm air flowing on exhalation from tube, condensate in tube, appropriate depth marking (at teeth)
Chest Radiograph (CXR)	A chest radiograph is a follow-up step for verifying proper tube position

End-tidal CO₂ Detector (P$_{ET}$CO$_2$) for Verification

CO$_2$ Detected (Yellow is YES)	
Tube likely in Trachea	Initial confirmation - verify with other methods. Most turn YELLOW.
CO$_2$ Not Detected (Purple is PROBLEM)	
Tube is in Esophagus	• Absent Chest Rise • Absent Breath Sounds • Stomach gurgling and distension
Tube is in Trachea *Verify with several other methods*	*Decreased CO$_2$ in Lungs:* • Poor blood flow to lungs • Cardiac arrest • Pulmonary embolus • IV bolus of epinephrine *Decreased CO$_2$ FROM Lungs:* • Airway obstruct (Status Asthmaticus, etc.) • Pulmonary edema • Mucus plugging
Unclear Where Tube Is	Detector contaminated with gastric contents or acidic drug
ETCO$_2$ device applied incorrectly, Time	Many disposable devices require "activation" (such as by pulling of paper tab), and may req. a few ventilations to change color

Esophageal Detector Device for Verification

Syringe-Type plunger is attached to ET Tube.	
Able to Pull Back on Plunger	ET Tube likely in trachea (rigid structure of trachea allows for air passage)
Unable to Pull Back on Plunger	ET Tube likely in esophagus (floppy structure of esophagus collapses over end of ET tube)
Caution: May be misleading in morbid obesity, late pregnancy, status asthmaticus, or with copious secretions. Use in children only if > 20 kg with perfusing rhythm.	

Tracheostomy Tubes
Types:

Characteristics	Typical Variations Available
Material	Metal (Jackson) Plastic (Shiley, Portex, Bivona, etc.)
Presence of Cuff	Cuffed or Uncuffed
Type of Cuff	Air, Fluid, or Foam Filled
Shape	Normal versus Specialty (extra-long: distal or proximal; custom)
Fenestrations	Fenestrated or Non-fenestrated
Inner Cannula	None or Removable (Non-disposable, Disposable)
Adjuncts	Speaking Valves (see next page)
Sizes	Vary, Adult usually 4-9

Indications for Tracheostomy Placement
- Patients unable to protect their airways
- Excessive secretions or can't maintain otherwise
- Swallowing or cough impairment with chronic aspiration
- Requiring invasive ventilation for a prolonged period
- Contraindications to, failed, or cannot tolerate NPPV
- Need to reduce anatomical dead space

Tracheostomy Care and Monitoring

- Basic vitals should be monitored (HR, RR, SpO$_2$)
- Humidity is usually required (upper airway is bypassed)
- Active humidity is recommended for new tracheostomies
- HMEs (passive humidity) are acceptable unless thick secretions, high minute ventilation, etc.
- Suctioning is preferably done when indicated (only): ensure trach-length in-line suction catheter is used
- There is evidence to support the use of trach bundles, protocol-directed care, and dedicated tracheostomy teams (AARC Clinical Practice Guideline, 2021)

Speaking Valves

Description	- A one-way valve placed on the trach tube
	  - Inhale: air comes in through valve
	  - Exhale: air is blocked from trach, goes through upper airway around trach

Purposes	- Enables verbal communication - Facilitates swallowing (eating/drinking) - Improves secretion clearance (cough secretions to upper airway)
Procedure	- **DEFLATE TRACH CUFF*** - Attach speaking valve to tracheostomy - If needed, increase V$_T$ on patients who are ventilator-dependent (leak has been created) - On initial placement, monitor for tolerance: vital signs, dyspnea, work of breathing - If indicated provide oxygen (over stoma)
Problems	- Air-trapping - Fatigue and/or intolerance - Mucus can occlude one-way valve

*Failing to deflate the cuff will result in the patient being able to inhale through the valve, but will have no way to exhale.

Tracheostomy Troubleshooting

Guiding Principles:
- Newly placed tracheostomies should be considered critical airways. If the trach comes out, it may be difficult to place back (or is more likely to go into a false tract)
- If the patient is in distress and the cause is the airway, remove the inner cannula. If no improvement, remove airway.
- To verify patency: run a suction catheter gently into the trach. If resistance is met, trach is either occluded (mucus, etc.) or is in soft tissue. Remove and check inner cannula.
- If unable to reinsert a trach, multiple options are available:
  - Cover stoma with gloved hand and use upper airway for BVM or intubation (if complete laryngectomy, do not use upper airway as there is no anatomical connection between upper and lower airways)
  - If stoma is patent, use a #6.0 ET tube (or smaller), insert several centimeters beyond stoma, then inflate cuff

Complications and Possible Actions

Complication	Possible Causes	Possible Actions
Cuff won't stay inflated	Cuff not patent (cuff leak evident)	Consider trach change, clamp pilot balloon line
Bleeding (from trach)	Suction trauma Blood from procedure Other causes	If small amount: monitor If new/large amount: notify physician
Chest pain	Cardiac Malpositioned trach Occluded trach Respiratory failure	Perform ECG (rule out cardiac) Verify placement (run suction catheter into tracheostomy to ensure no occlusion) Discontinue capping trial
Crackling/edema around stoma	Trach in soft tissue (crepitus)	Verify placement Consider trach change

Complication	Possible Causes	Possible Actions
High cuff pressures to seal Should be 20-25 mmHg	Incorrect size	Consider trach change (Note: increasing trach size is challenging, ensure adequate support)
Difficulty passing suction catheter	Suction catheter too large Malpositioned trach Occluded trach	**Consider lavage. If still unable to pass suction catheter, and/or patient distress, remove and inspect inner cannula. If still unable to pass catheter, likely need to remove the trach.**
Excessive secretions, Change in secretions	Infection Humidity (excess) Humidity (insufficient)	Send sputum culture Check labs See pg 4-16 for secretions Consider humidity setting (heat may liquefy secretions, turn down temp if clinically appropriate) If thick secretions, consider change from HME (if used) to active humidity
Skin redness Drainage (Pus)	Infection Pressure wound	Culture if infection suspected Consider cleaning with 1:1 mixture of Hydrogen Peroxide with NS*
Granulation Tissue (immature blood vessels, may cause bleeding to occur easily)	Extended placement	Consider regular trach changes (every 1-2 weeks)
Excessive coughing or gagging, dyspnea, feeling of choking	Excessive secretions Tolerance of trach	Non-pharmacological or pharmacological airway clearance Anxiety interventions

*Hydrogen peroxide may be irritating and is not recommended for routine cleaning, but may help with infected skin/stoma

Tracheostomy Daily Care

1. Explain procedure to patient
2. Position patient supine or head slightly elevated
3. Stand to side of patient (pt is likely to cough)
4. Perform hand hygiene, don gloves, face shield/mask
5. Gently clean stoma with normal saline (or sterile water), noting skin integrity and secretions
6. Replace inner cannula, trach tie, gauze/dressing, taking care to secure the tracheostomy tube at all times

Performing a Tracheostomy Change
A second skilled person should be at the bedside to assist with the trach change

1. Explain procedure to patient
2. Position patient supine (sniffing position) or slightly elevated
3. Perform hand hygiene, don gloves, face shield/mask
4. Clean stoma from inner to outer rim (use normal saline or sterile water), then dry
5. Remove inner cannula of new tube (if present), insert obturator. Check new cuff for leaks (if cuffed).
6. Lubricate outside of tube with water-soluble lubricant
7. Stand on side of pt to avoid exposure to body fluids from trach (patient is likely to cough)
8. Oxygenate, suction trach and airway, re-oxygenate
9. Remove holder/tie, have patient take a deep breath (or give deep breath with resuscitation bag), <u>deflate cuff</u>, then remove old trach tube gently
10. Quickly, but gently, insert new tube (sideways, then gently downward) (do not force), hold tube in place and immediately remove obturator
11. Insert inner cannula and lock in place (if present), inflate cuff, if present
12. Verify placement ($ETCO_2$, pass suction catheter, auscultate, feel for air flow). Remove tube if cannot be placed properly or airflow is inadequate; ventilate as needed and attempt to reinsert tube.
13. Hold tube in place until urge to cough subsides
14. Secure trach holder/ties (leave one finger width loose)
15. Suction and oxygenate if needed. Re-auscultate/assess.

Non-disposable Tracheostomy Tube/Inner Cannula

1. Perform hand hygiene, don gloves, face shield/mask
2. Open all packages
3. Suction tracheostomy tube before removing
4. Remove inner cannula by unlocking/gently pulling outward or remove single tube or outer cannula by cutting ties, holding tube in place with finger, deflate cuff, pull gently outward and downward
5. Soak tube in cleaning solution for indicated time
6. Clean skin/stoma with cotton dipped in solution and pat dry with gauze
7. Brush inside of tube with cleaning solution
8. Rinse tube thoroughly with sterile water
9. Pat dry with clean gauze and replace

Considerations for Trach Changes

Variable	Considerations
Equipment	Always have a BVM ready and connected to O_2 with appropriate flow running. Intubation equip. should be easily accessible.
People at Bedside	Minimum of 2 qualified people
Age of Trach	Fresh tracheostomies (< 1 week old) should be changed only if emergent, and by MD. Risk of loss of patent airway if pulled. Intubation equipment should be present.
Anatomical	**Caution Should be Used in:** • Obese Patients • Abnormal neck anatomy • Any trach placed for patency
Size	Downsizing is generally easier than replacing same size: use caution in upsizing
Verification	Always verify correct placement following a trach change. Use auscultation, $ETCO_2$, chest rise, return volumes if on vent, SpO_2, WOB, ability to pass suction catheter and/or able to "bag" patient effectively

Tracheostomy Capping and Decannulation Trials[1]

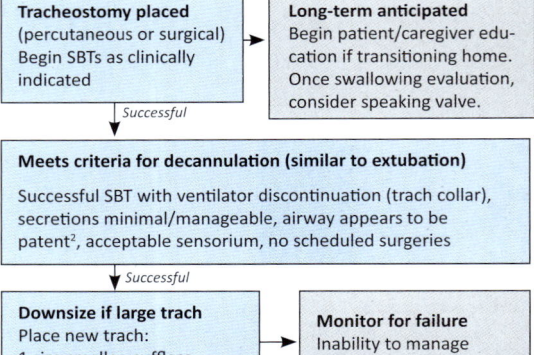

[1] Consistent with AAO-HNS Consensus Guidelines
[2] Swallow evaluation and/or endoscopic assessment if concerns
[3] If cuffed trach, ensure it is deflated for capping trial

Ventilation Management

Improving Ventilation: $PaCO_2$ (and pH)	
Goal	Maintain adequate CO_2 elimination while protecting the lungs from injury.
Principle	Adequacy of ventilation is mostly determined by minute ventilation, and assessed by $PaCO_2$/pH (Several therapeutic strategies exist, including lung protection) (see Permissive Hypercapnia)
	$PaCO_2$ and resultant pH are impacted by total ventilation, deadspace, and CO_2 production. They are changed by altering minute ventilation, deadspace and/or CO_2 production. Note that deadspace is not often used therapeutically anymore.

Estimate to achieve a desired $PaCO_2$ using:	Equation
Minute Ventilation	$\text{New } \dot{V}_E = \dfrac{\text{Current } \dot{V}_E \times \text{Current } PaCO_2}{\text{Desired } PaCO_2}$
Tidal Volume	$\text{New } V_T = \dfrac{\text{Current } V_T \times \text{Current } PaCO_2}{\text{Desired } PaCO_2}$
Set Rate	$\text{New } f = \dfrac{\text{Current } f \times \text{Current } PaCO_2}{\text{Desired } PaCO_2}$

These equations assume a patient is on a control-mode of ventilation, not making spontaneous efforts. The formulas can be used only as an estimate in spontaneously breathing patients.

Management

Acute Respiratory Acidosis
↑ $PaCO_2$ with ↓ pH (inadequate minute ventilation)

Strategy: ensure optimized V/Q, then increase minute ventilation

Mode Type	Primary Strategies
Volume	1. Increase f (be sure to adjust T_I simultaneously to ensure adequate exhalation). 2. Increase V_T - use with caution! Most of the time V_T is set by mL/kg IBW, so it is less common to increase V_T. (see page 7-15 for calculations)
Pressure	1. Increase f (be sure to adjust T_I simultaneously to ensure adequate exhalation). 2. Increase V_T by either increasing Inspiratory Pressure, or increasing T_I. Again, use with caution as V_T is most often set by mL/kg IBW, so it is less common to increase V_T. (see page 7-15 for calculations)

Additional Strategies

Increase spontaneous tidal volume
- Add or increase pressure support to spontaneous breaths
- Ensure appropriate airway clearance/bronchodilation
- Exchange ET tube for larger tube
- Ensure adequate muscle conditioning, nutrition

Decrease mechanical deadspace (uncommon)
- Consider circuit compliance, ET tube length
- Tracheostomy tube (vs endotracheal tube)

Consider high-frequency ventilation

Allow for permissive hypercapnia

↑ PaCO₂ with ↓ pH (adequate/high minute ventilation)

Strategy: identify potential causes, treat (see table below)

Potential Causes	Strategies
↑ **Deadspace (VD/VT)**	
Air trapping	Ensure adequate TE
High I:E Ratio	Ensure adequate TE (decrease I:E)
Uneven gas distribution (V/Q)	Recruit with PEEP/mPAW Place bad lung up (unilateral) Place in prone (bilateral)
Pulmonary embolus	Verify (CT scan, etc.) and treat PE
↑ **CO₂ Production**	
Stress (trauma, surgery)	Increase minute ventilation (ensure no auto-PEEP)
Fever	Treat fever
Burns	Increase minute ventilation (ensure no auto-PEEP) Consider APRV (TCAV), HFPV
Sepsis	Treat underlying sepsis Use lung protective strategies (allow for hypercapnia)

APRV: Airway Pressure Release Ventilation (see page 3-20)
HFPV: High-Frequency Percussive Ventilation

Management

Acute Respiratory Alkalosis
↓ $PaCO_2$ and ↑ pH
If underlying hypoxemia, treat that first

Note: A respiratory alkalosis present in patients "riding the vent" (Total RR = Set RR) is clinician-induced and should be corrected. A Respiratory Alkalosis in a patient who has spontaneous breaths must be further analyzed before fixing - alkalosis in this case is sometimes left uncorrected

Mode Type	Strategies
Volume	1. Decrease f. See Quick Formula on previous page for calculating f. 2. Decrease V_T - when V_T > Deadspace Ventilation
Pressure	1. Decrease f 2. Decrease V_T by either decreasing Inspiratory Pressure, or carefully decreasing T_I. Again, use with caution as V_T is most often set by mL/kg IBW, so it is less common to increase V_T. (see page 7-15 for calculations)

Additional Strategies

Trial spontaneous mode of ventilation (patient has more control)

Consider increase of sedation (if severe agitation, anxiety, pain, or associated with increased work of breathing/asynchrony)

Add VD_{mech} (not often used clinically)

Metabolic Disorders

Under normal physiology, the lungs will nearly instantly compensate for an abnormal metabolic state. This might not be the case if:
- Severe metabolic acidosis or alkalosis (unable to compensate)
- Sedation or vent settings (patient is fully dependent on vent)
- Underlying pathophysiology (COPD, etc.)
- Respiratory failure (patient has tired, for example)

Ventilator Settings
Treating the underlying cause of the metabolic dysfunction is usually most effective but not always attainable. Ventilator settings (primarily the rate) can be used to manipulate the pH, to a point.

Metabolic Acidosis
↓ HCO_3 with ↓ $PaCO_2$, normal or ↓ pH
Compensation: high minute ventilation (hyperventilating)

- Correct the cause of the metabolic acidosis when possible and known
- Increase the set rate when significant acidosis (increase vent breaths, increase or add PS if V_T is appropriate)
- Consider admin of sodium bicarb when life-threatening acidosis

Metabolic Alkalosis
↑ HCO_3 with ↑ $PaCO_2$, normal or ↑ pH
Compensation: low minute ventilation (hypoventilating)

- Correct the cause of the metabolic acidosis when possible and known
- Decrease the set rate when significant alkalosis (decrease vent breaths if patient is matching vent rate, cautiously decrease PS - watch for WOB)
- Consider sedation/paralytics if severe alkalosis and patient is driving the ventilator rate above expected

Permissive Hypercapnia	
Definition	Therapeutically allowing the CO_2 to increase (and thus pH to drop to acidosis) by limiting ventilatory support - usually VT
Goal	Lung protection (prevent damage to alveoli)
Indications	Many clinicians employ permissive hypercapnia in the majority of critical care patients (prophylactic) Any time Pplat is rising (close to 30 cmH$_2$O)
Contraindications (Relative)	Cerebral traumas, hemorrhage, CNS lesions ($\uparrow CO_2 \rightarrow$ cerebral vasodilation $\rightarrow \uparrow$ ICP) and CV instability ($\uparrow PaCO_2$ and $\downarrow$ pH may lead to $\downarrow$ myocardial contractility, arrhythmias, and/or vasodilation)
How To	Ventilate with low VT (4-7 mL/kg IBW) to keep Pplat ≤ 30 cmH$_2$O. 4 mL is lower end of VT range due to anatomic deadspace of around 2 mL/kg IBW $PaCO_2$ is allowed to $\uparrow$ to 50 - 100 mmHg and pH is allowed to $\downarrow$ to 7.15 - 7.20. Introduction of hypercapnia should be gradual (< 10 mmHg/hr)
Considerations	Patients may require increased sedation to tolerate lower VT strategy PEEP should be optimized to maintain lung recruitment with lower VT. Consider Sodium Bicarbonate or other intervention for patients with pH < 7.15
Physiologic Effects	CNS depression, May $\uparrow$ ICP. May reduce PaO_2, Right shift of oxyhemoglobin curve, dyspnea (stimulation of ventilation), pulmonary vasoconstriction, CV effects (hypotension)

Management

Oxygenation

Improving Oxygenation: PaO₂ (SaO₂, SpO₂)	
Goal	To maintain adequate O_2 delivery to the tissues while ventilating with the lowest possible F_iO_2 and pressures.
Principle	PaO_2 is affected primarily by F_iO_2, $\overline{Paw}$ (V_T, PIP, PEEP, T_I, $\dot{V}I$, $\dot{V}I$ waveform) and cardiovascular disease (i.e., optimizing lung volume and V/Q matching). Adequate O_2 delivery to tissues is dependent on F_iO_2, cardiac output, and CaO_2.

Quick Estimates of Oxygenation Status:

P/F ratio = PaO_2/F_iO_2
- PaO_2 is the amount of oxygen in the arteries
- F_iO_2 is the amount of oxygen in the alveoli (roughly, of course)
- The ratio estimates how well oxygen is getting from alveoli to the arteries.
- Normal is approximately 500

S/F ratio = SpO_2/F_iO_2
- Values are equivalent to P/F but achieved noninvasively
- Assumed adequate peripheral perfusion

Oxygen Index (OI) = $\dfrac{F_iO_2 \times \overline{Paw} \times 100}{PaO_2}$ F_iO_2 is a decimal

OI again estimates the amount of oxygen that goes from alveoli to blood, but takes into account mean airway pressure, which we know is greatly impacted by factors like PEEP. Thus, the OI can be considered a more powerful estimate of oxygenation.

Strategies for Improving Oxygenation

See following pages for further explanations. FIO₂ is often the first method utilized, but comes with its own hazards (see pg 10-8), and so other methods should then be used to wean the FIO₂ to a safer level.

Strategy	How It Contributes
Increase FIO$_2$ pg 7-23	• Increases the O$_2$ tension/gradient (more O$_2$ is potentially available) • Ineffective when there is refractory hypoxemia (ARDS, COVID, etc.)
Optimize PEEP pg 7-24	• Optimizes functional residual capacity (assuming no underlying auto-PEEP) • Contributes to mPAW (increases FRC) • Decreases shunting
Optimize mPAW pg 7-32	• Optimizes functional residual capacity (FRC)
Optimize Positioning pg 7-33	• Works to better match ventilation with perfusion (good ventilation with good perfusion, and minimize ventilation where there is an absence of good perfusion) • Use of either modified position (unilateral processes) or proning (bilateral processes)
Consider Inverse Ratio Ventilation pg 7-36	• Optimizes functional residual capacity (FRC) • Employed by manipulating the I:E ratio (less common) or using a mode that incorporates IRV (APRV, for example)

1. FiO₂	
Goal	Use the minimum amount of supplemental oxygen necessary to maintain <u>adequate</u> oxygenation (not necessarily normal oxygenation)
Principle	This is a major determinant of oxygenation, increasing the $P(A-a)O_2$ gradient, which usually results in a greater PaO_2.
Clinical Notes	• Increase FiO_2 incrementally • Clinically, increasing FiO_2 initially in response to acute distress is appropriate. • Higher FiO_2 over time increases the risk of hyperoxic lung injury so the overall goal is to maintain < 0.50 when possible with conservative PaO_2 goals around 60-80 torr

Calculating FiO₂ to alter PaO₂
New FiO₂ = $\dfrac{\text{Desired PaO}_2 \times \text{Known FiO}_2}{\text{Known PaO}_2}$

2. PEEP	
Goal	OPTIMAL PEEP which: ↑ **PaO$_2$** – ↓ shunt effect, ↑ FRC, and ↑ C, allowing for the reduction of FiO$_2$ and its complications. ↓ **WOB** – Unload the inspiratory muscles (esp. in acute exacerbation of COPD).
Principle	Determinant of oxygenation by affecting Paw.
Clinical Notes	Maintains pressures above ambient pressure during the expiratory phase to prevent collapse of smaller airways and unstable alveoli.
Contra-indications	**Absolute**: Tension Pneumothorax Untreated Pneumothorax (significant in size) **Relative**: - Barotrauma - Bronchopulmonary fistula - Pre-existing hyperinflation (COPD, etc.) - Hypovolemia - Recent lung surgery - Unilateral lung disorders
Beneficial Effects	- Increased mPAW - Increased compliance - Increased PaO$_2$ - Decreased WOB - Increased preload/afterload (some heart failure patients may benefit) - Increased V/Q (improves gas distribution and ↓ right-to-left shunting) - Increased functional residual capacity
Adverse Effects	- Alveolar overdistension (leads to volutrauma) - Increased WOB - Increased V$_D$/V$_T$ (pulm. capillary compression) - Cardiovascular effects (dependent on PEEP level, compliance, and cardiovascular status)

Initiate PEEP/CPAP Therapy

1. Increase PEEP incrementally if not performing Optimal PEEP maneuver (see below) - usually by 3-5 cmH₂O every 10-15 minutes
2. Monitor patient carefully for response
   - desired response (optimization): improvement in O₂ without hemodynamic deterioration
   - undesired response (likely alveolar overdistension): hemodynamic compromise (hypotension, bradycardia), usually without O₂ improvement
3. Periodically reassess acid-base, oxygenation indices, ventilation, respiratory mechanics, and hemodynamic parameters.

PEEP Ranges*

PEEP Level	Range (cmH₂O)	Clinical Intention
Low	3-7	Match physiologic PEEP lost when bypassing vocal cords. This preserves the FRC.
Moderate	8-10	Treat refractory hypoxemia caused by ↑ intrapulmonary shunting with ↓ FRC and ↓ C.
High	> 10	Use may be indicated with severe shunting or external pressures (obesity, etc.). Increased risk of overdistension (hemodynamic compromise).
Optimal PEEP	determined clinically	the level of PEEP at which oxygen delivery to the tissues is maximized. See next page

*These PEEP ranges are rather arbitrary. The ranges are meant to illustrate clinical intention (rather than be an exact range). Optimal PEEP is preferred.

Methods for Determining Optimal PEEP

1. **Incremental PEEP Study**
   - Increase PEEP by about 3 cmH$_2$O at a time, calculating static compliance (inspiratory hold) at each step.
   $C_{stat} = V_T/(P_{plat} - PEEP)$
   - Use the level of applied PEEP that resulted in the best compliance (largest C_{stat})

   Alternative: Increase PEEP by 2-3 cmH$_2$O at a time, carefully observing SpO$_2$, V$_T$, and BP. Optimal PEEP is determined to be the minimum PEEP which increases V$_T$ and potentially SpO$_2$ without causing a decrease in BP (suggesting you are over-distending).

2. **PEEP/F$_I$O$_2$ tables** (ARDSnet) See ARDS, page 9-2

3. **Use P-V loop**
   Preferred: Use the ventilator's tool, when available, for setting PEEP
   - Set PEEP between the lower inflection point and upper inflection point (see diagram on next page)
   - Consider administration of a dose of heavy sedation with or without a paralytic in order to obtain accurate P-V loop
   - Identify lower and upper inflection points (LIP and UIP) on loop

4. **Oxygenation PEEP Study**
   - A goal PaO$_2$ is set (60 torr, for example)
   - PEEP is titrated over a period of time to achieve the target PaO$_2$ with an F$_I$O$_2$ < 0.50

5. **Esophageal Pressure**
   - Balloon catheter is placed in esophagus which is used to estimate pleural pressure
   - Transpulmonary Pressure = P$_{aw}$ - P$_{pleural}$
   Goal: End-inspiratory Transpulmonary Pressure < 25 cmH$_2$O

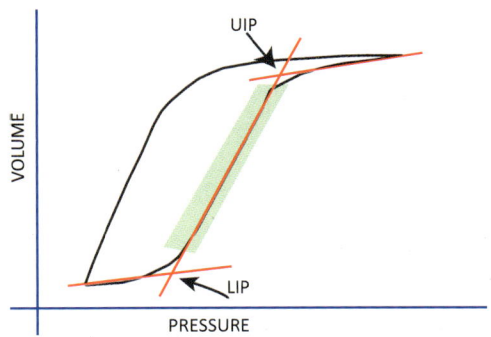

Understanding the P-V Loop and PEEP:
1. The steep part of the curve represents rapid increases in volume with small pressure changes, implying best compliance as the lungs accept volume easily.
2. The flattened sections represent areas where it takes greater pressures to move small volumes of air (the cost of ventilation, and the risk of lung damage, is high):
   Lower: Lower flattened section suggests areas of the lungs that are closing and opening, which results in atelectrauma. These are separated in the above diagram by the lower inflection point (LIP).
   Upper: Upper flattened section ("duckbill"), when present, suggests over-distension, which can lead to barotrauma (damage caused by excessive pressure). PEEP should always be set below the upper inflection point (UIP).
3. The slope of the curve provides information about lung compliance. Less steep curves suggest poor compliance (it always takes a fair amount of pressure to deliver a volume)
4. Ideally this curve is captured with no patient contribution, meaning it is most accurate when a patient is given a single-dose of a paralytic. Note that the LIP in particular is not always discernible.

Other Approaches to Setting PEEP*

By Chest Radiograph

Chest Radiograph Appearance	Suggested Starting PEEP (cmH_2O)
Clear	5
Diffuse Infiltrates	10
Dense Infiltrates	15
Bilateral Whiteout	20

By P/F Ratio

P/F Ratio	Suggested Starting PEEP (cmH_2O)
> 200	5-10
> 100	10-15
≤ 100	15-20

*Based in part on Owens W. The Ventilator Book. 3rd editon (2021); First Draught Press

Using Applied PEEP in the presence of Auto-PEEP

Applied PEEP (extrinsic PEEP) may be applied up to 80% of measured auto-PEEP. This technique is specifically for patients who have an expiratory flow limitation (prevents airways collapse during exhalation)

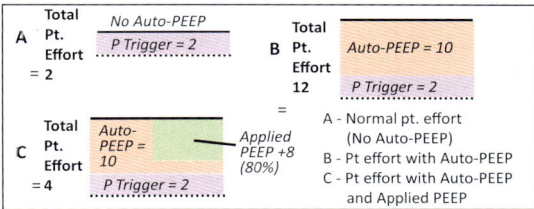

A - Normal pt. effort (No Auto-PEEP)
B - Pt effort with Auto-PEEP
C - Pt effort with Auto-PEEP and Applied PEEP

It is thought that up to 80% of applied PEEP only affects the circuit and airway pressures and not alveolar pressures. It works to equilibrate trapped pressure and circuit pressure.

Applied PEEP should be kept less than auto-PEEP (< 80%, some clinicians recommend < 50%) as at higher amounts alveolar pressures will increase, which will increase risk of adverse effects (barotrauma, cardiovascular compromise). Use the lowest required PEEP to accomplish triggering.

Techniques for Setting Appropriate Applied PEEP
1. Incremental approach: increase PEEP in increments of 2-5 cmH$_2$O until the patient can reliably trigger a ventilator breath (a slight deflection in pressure should be followed by a breath)
2. Esophageal balloon: may help estimate pleural pressures (alveolar pressures need to be higher than pleural pressures to prevent end-expiratory collapse)

Parameters for Assessing PEEP

These assessments should be considered within the context of PEEP being insufficient (too low) or excessive (too high). In general: there should be an improvement in oxygenation and ventilation as PEEP is optimized (titrated higher), beyond which parameters deteriorate (overdistension)

Assessing Oxygenation (PEEP)

Parameter	Goal
FIO_2	Weaning to < 0.50
PaO_2 SaO_2	Improving or steady with FIO_2 weaning
P/F Ratio	Increasing (> 300)
$P(A-a)O_2$	Decreasing
Q_S/Q_T	Decreasing

Assessing Ventilation (PEEP)

Parameter	Goal
Breath Sounds	Improving aeration (recruitment)
Driving Pressure	Decreasing
PIP	Decreasing towards normal
Pplat	Decreasing towards normal
Cdyn	Increasing towards normal
Cstat	Increasing towards normal
Raw	Decreasing towards normal
Acid-Base	Improvement in pH, $PaCO_2$ if recruitment

Assessing Hemodynamics (PEEP)

Parameter	Goal
Blood Pressure	Adequate, up to 20% decrease
Cardiac Output	Adequate, up to 20% decrease
PA Pressures	Towards normal
PCWP	Stable Marked Increase: overdistension? Marked decrease: ↓ CO?
$P\bar{v}O_2$	Increasing, > 28 mmHg
$S\bar{v}O_2$	Increasing, > 50%
$C(a-\bar{v})O_2$	Decreasing

Considerations in Weaning PEEP

- Consider weaning once Pplat < 30 cmH$_2$O and FiO$_2$ < 0.50
- Use a gradual approach unless hemodynamic compromise: decrease by 1-2 cmH$_2$O every 1-6 hours
- If PaO$_2$ decreases by > 20% (consider other relevant parameters as well: P/F, driving pressure, etc.) after a weaning step, increase to the previous level
- Goal is to wean to a baseline PEEP, somewhere around 5 cmH$_2$O (though there are exceptions with certain diseases/disorders, when a higher baseline PEEP may be indicated)

3. Mean Airway Pressure (mPAW, $\overline{Paw}$, or MAP)	
Goal	Achieve adequate oxygenation with the lowest possible pressures and FiO₂ without impairing cardiovascular function or injuring the lungs
Principle	mPAW is an important determinant/reflection of oxygenation. It is primarily determined by PIP, PEEP, and Inspiratory Time (TI).
Indication	Consider increasing mPAW in patients with low lung volumes and evidence of refractory hypoxemia ($PaO_2 < 60$ torr on $FIO_2 > 0.6$)
Potential Risks of ↑ mPAW	*(when overdistension occurs)* Barotrauma Decreased cardiac output

Calculation of Mean Airway Pressure

Most often mPAW is automatically calculated by the ventilator. This may not include any auto-PEEP.

Type of Ventilation	Calculation mPAW=
Volume Ventilation (constant flow)	$0.5 \times (PIP - PEEP) \times (T_I / T_{total}) + PEEP$
Pressure Ventilation	$(PIP - PEEP) \times (T_I / T_{total}) + PEEP$

* The mean alveolar pressure may be different than mPAW if there are differences between inspiratory and expiratory airway resistance

4. Patient Positioning
Proning technique and considerations are on the following pages

Goal	Improve V/Q and FRC by placing patient in various positions - usually either lateral (right side down or left side down) or by proning patient (chest-side down)
Principle	Attempts to optimize gas exchange by aligning perfusion (blood is partially gravity-dependent) with ventilation (placing the more compliant/healthy lung regions where the better perfusion is). **Modified Position:** *Unilateral processes (pneumonia, etc.)* Bad Lung UP, Good Lung DOWN (can be remembered as BLU GLD ... Blue Gold) Exception: pulmonary hemorrhage, lung abscess, etc. (place in opposite position of above) **Proned Position:** *Bilateral processes (ARDS, COVID, etc.)* Patient is placed chest-side down in bed See considerations and procedures on the following pages
Clinical Notes	• Consider contraindications prior to positioning (trauma, cardiovascular compromise, c-spine instability) • Monitor patient carefully for deterioration, ventilator trends/parameters, complications, etc • Some level of improvement is most likely within 30-60 minutes • Assessing for response is similar to assessing PEEP (see page 7-30)

Management

Proning Procedure (Respiratory Considerations):

Verify no contraindications *Consider other techniques or modified positioning if contraindications*	• Increased ICP (clear with neuro) • Massive hemoptysis • Tracheostomy • Facial trauma (including eyes) • C-spine injury (unstable) • Pregnancy • Open abdomen
Ensure adequate team members at bedside	Minimum of 3 people needed (1 for airway, 1 on each side of bed) Consider additional staff as indicated (morbid obesity, complex devices/lines/tube, etc.)
Consider safety	Respiratory therapist at head of bed should guide process (start, speed) using standard language ("Is everyone ready? On my count we turn after 3.").
Place patient on side	• Take note of ET tube position/depth • Turn patient to one side, securing airway and neck/spine. • Patient should be moved to side of bed away from the ventilator (allows for slack with ventilator circuit) • Pause to allow for reposition of both ECG leads (to patient's back) and lines/tubes (above waist towards head of bed, below waist towards foot of bed)
Place patient prone	Turn patient prone (slowly), supporting the ET tube and neck alignment. Head may be on side (facing ventilator initially) or down (if device available).
Verify	• ET tube depth/position, kinks • Cuff leak • Areas of pressure around ET tube • Breath sounds • Ventilator parameters

Proning Management (Respiratory Considerations)

Ventilator Assessments	- Lung V/Q will be altered. Watch pulmonary mechanics and adjust ventilator parameters as indicated. - Goal: improvement in oxygenation (P/F ratio, etc.) with stable or improving ventilation.
Artificial Airway Assessments	- It may be necessary to add air to the ET tube cuff initially. The frequent need to add air may indicate a problem and needs to be evaluated - The head should be repositioned every few hours. Ensure airway patency and position each time
Skin Integrity Assessments	- Due to gravity, dependent areas may become edematous, especially the face - Carefully and regularly assess edema/stress around the ET tube and the ET tube stabilization device. - Consider clinical appropriateness of device being utilized

5. Inverse Ratio Ventilation (IRV) *Not typically used (as a mode) in current clinical practice*	
Goal	Setting I:E ratio with TI being greater than TE (I:E ratio > 1:1)
Principle	Increasing TI to increase mPAW and recruit and keep alveoli open for extended periods in order to improve V/Q without overinflating normal alveolar units
Indication	When conventional ventilator strategies with optimal PEEP have resulted in P_{plat} > 30 cmH$_2$O without providing an acceptable P/F ratio.
Risks	• Auto-PEEP (dynamic hyperinflation) • Increased PIP in volume-IRV • Decreased VT in pressure-IRV • Decreased V̇E (↓ VT or air-trapping) • Decreased cardiac output
Strategy	Increase TI in 0.1-0.2 sec increments until either P/F ratio goal is achieved or air-trapping develops. Sedation and paralytics may be required for tolerance of IRV Increase TI by: • Increasing inspiratory time • Decreasing inspiratory flow (volume modes) • Transition to decelerating flow pattern (volume does) • Institute an inspiratory pause (unusual)
Clinical Notes	• Some specialty modes (APRV, BiVent, BiLevel) are basically IRV, but allow for spontaneous breaths during the extended TI, which may improve synchrony. • Studies have not demonstrated any advantage of using IRV over other methods, but risks are greater (Auto-PEEP, ↑ PIP, ↓ CO, ↓ synchrony)

Airway Clearance Management

Suctioning

Guiding principles of suctioning:
- Perform when indicated, not as a scheduled procedure
- Attempts should be kept to a duration of 15 seconds or less
- Due to its invasive nature, this is a preferred sterile procedure, minimally a "clean" procedure
- Use the lowest effective pressure (see next page for suction pressures)
- Types of Suction
  - Open: advancing a suction catheter into the airway (natural or artificial)
  - Closed (also called in-line): a suction catheter within a sheath keeps a circuit "closed" (if on a ventilator), goal is to minimize risk of ventilator-associated pneumonia (VAP)

Indications/Need

Evidence of Secretions	• Visible secretions in artificial airway • Auscultation: coarse crackles, decreased • Palpation: coarse vibrations
Alterations in Patient/ Ventilator Interaction	• Patient: ↑ agitation, irritability, restlessness • Ventilator: ↑ Raw Volume Mode: ↑ PIP, High Pressure alarm Pressure Mode: ↓ V$_T$
Alterations in Vital Signs	• Change in respiratory pattern: ↑ WOB, tachypnea, retractions • Change in cardiac pattern: ↑ or ↓ HR
Alterations in O$_2$ and Ventilation	• ↓ SpO$_2$: often trends steadily but may drop quickly, particularly if a mucous plug • Skin color: pale, dusky, or cyanotic • ABG: ↓ PaO$_2$, respiratory acidosis

Suction Pressures for Airways

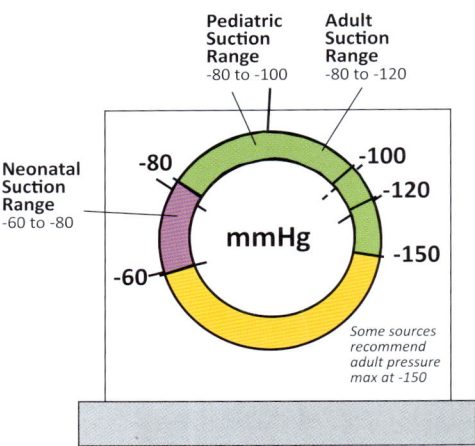

Suction Catheter Sizing

Suction catheter should be < 50% of the internal diameter of the ET Tube (but large enough to suction thicker sputum, mucous plugs, etc.).

Suction Catheter Size (FR) = (ET Tube Size x 3) / 2
(if not an even number, drop to next smallest even number)

Example:
Pt with a size 7.5 cm ET Tube
= (7.5 x 3) / 2
= 22.5/2
= 11.25
Next Smallest = 10 FR

High Frequency Oscillations (HFO) Summary

See following pages for detailed information on devices

Airway Oscillations

Patient Generated	*Oscillatory PEP Therapy*	The patient's active exhalation through a device performs the work of creating oscillations which are transferred to the patient's airway.
	*For use off a ventilator (adapted with a trach), but can't be used with a ventilator*	
Device Generated	*Intrapulmonary Percussive Ventilation (IPV)*	A device which creates short, rapid inspiratory flow pulses into the airway. Expiration is passive from chest wall elastic recoil.
	Ex: MetaNeb, Percussionator, PercussiveNeb, IMP2	

Chest Wall Oscillations

Device Generated	*High Frequency Chest Wall Compression (HFCWC)* *Vest/Cuirass*	A device which creates short, rapid expiratory flow pulses in the airway by compressing the chest wall externally. Chest wall elastic recoil returns lung to FRC.
	Ex: The Vest, SmartVest, InCourage	
	High Frequency Chest Wall Oscillation (HFCWO)	A device which creates short, rapid biphasic (positive + negative) pressure changes (oscillations) on the chest wall externally, which is transferred to the airway.
	Ex: Hayek Oscillator	

Intrapulmonary Percussive Ventilation (IPV)	
Description	The delivery of high-frequency percussive breaths (sub-tidal volume) into the patient's airways by a pneumatic device.
Indications	The inability to effectively cough or clear secretions as a result of reduced peak expiratory flow rates.
Contraindications	Bronchospasm, lung contusion, pneumothorax, pulmonary hemorrhage, subcutaneous emphysema, TB, vomiting and aspiration.
Directions	• Pt breathes through a mouthpiece or artificial airway and the unit delivers high flow rate bursts of gas into the lungs from 100-300/min. Continuous positive pressure is maintained (typically 15-40 cm H_2O) while the pulses dilate the airways. At the end of the percussive inspiratory cycle (5-10 sec), a deep exhalation is performed with expectoration of secretions. • Normal treatment time is 20 min. Aerosols (bland or medicated) may also be delivered via the attached nebulizer.
Settings	• Pressure is set via a manometer with optimum range being 30-40 cmH_2O (less for ↑ Compliance, more for ↓ Compliance). This is equivalent to setting a "mean airway pressure" • Difficulty knob changes the frequency of the oscillations which may improve clearance and recruitment. It is recommended that this knob be turned back and forth every few minutes during treatment.
Notes	• Can be performed with mechanical ventilation • Circuit configurations are different for ventilator versus non-vented, and should be assembled carefully • When effective, several breaks may need to be taken in order to get pt to cough or suction. • Many clinicians recommend utilizing an in-line suction catheter when used in conjunction with an artificial airway to facilitate suctioning. • Cuffed artificial airways: Suction above cuff, and then at least partially deflate cuff during treatment to facilitate secretion clearance.

Percussive Vests/Wraps	
Description	• The system includes an air pulse generator, inflatable vest, and connecting tube. • It provides high frequency chest wall compressions which help mobilize secretions.
Indications	• Cystic fibrosis, bronchiectasis, or conditions where the patient is unable to effectively mobilize and expectorate secretions.
Contra-indications	Active hemorrhage, cardiac instability, chest wall pain, lung contusion, recent thoracic skin grafts, recently placed pacemaker, subcutaneous emphysema, suspected tuberculosis, unstable head and/or neck injury.
Directions	• As the patient wears the inflatable vest, small gas volumes alternately flow into and out of the unit – rapidly inflating and deflating (compressing and releasing) the chest wall to create air flow and cough- like shear forces to move secretions. • Timing of the pulse is manually controlled by the patient or clinician • The intensity (25-40 mmHg) and frequency (5-25 Hz) of the pulses can also be adjusted by the patient or clinician • Vests come in various styles (full chest vest down to simple wrap around chest), disposable/nondisposable, and sizes. Ensuring a proper fit and style helps ensure better pt compliance with therapy.

Humidity Management

Variable	Considerations
Indications	**Primary Indications** • Humidify dry medical gases (> 4 L/min) • Overcome humidity deficit when upper airway is bypassed **Secondary Indications** • Treat bronchospasm due to cold air • Treat hypothermia • Thickened secretions
Therapeutic Modalities	Used specifically with the following modalities: • Oxygen therapy with higher flow rates • Non-invasive positive pressure ventilation (CPAP and NPPV ventilation) • Invasive positive pressure ventilation • Artificial airways via collar or T-Piece
Under-Humidification	• Atelectasis (mucus plugging) • Dry, nonproductive cough • Substernal pain • Thick, dehydrated secretions • Hypoxemia • ↑ Airway resistance • ↑ Infection • ↑ WOB
Over-Humidification	• Fluid overload • Pulmonary edema • Surfactant alteration • Thermal damage to mucosa • ↑ Airway secretions (↑ airway resistance) • Atelectasis • Hypoxemia
Heat	• Heated humidification is recommended for artificial airways, thick secretions, and/or patient comfort

Heated Humidity

- Close monitoring of operating and output temperatures, adequate water supply/proper level, and condensation buildup is required
- Prevent inadvertent tracheal lavage from the condensate
- Check that alarms are set and working properly
- For targeted temperature management (induced hypothermia), evidence lacks. If turning off humidifier or using HME during hypothermia, monitor closely for deterioration related to dehydrated secretions, bronchoconstriction.

Humidification During Invasive and Noninvasive Mechanical Ventilation** (AARC Expert Reference-Based Guideline)

Indication
Mandatory with ET tube or Trach Tube.
Optional with NIV (use HH if humidifying)

Contraindication
None except **HME** when: Body temperature < 32°C, low V_T strategies, expired V_T < 70% of delivered V_T, spont $\dot{V}_E$ > 10 L/min, thick, copious, or bloody secretions.

Monitoring
Check: alarm settings (30 – 41°C) (HH), humidifier temp setting (HH), inspired gas temp (34-40°C) (HH), water level and feed system (HH), sputum quantity and consistency
Remove condensate in circuit, Replace HMEs contaminated with secretions

Frequency:
Continuous during gas therapy

Hazards/Complications
Burns (patient or caregiver)(HH)
Electrical shock (HH)
Hypo/hyperthermia
Hypoventilation (HME → ↑V_D)
↑ Resistive WOB through humidifier
Infection (nosocomial)
Tracheal lavage (pooled condensate or overfilling) (HH)
Underhydration (mucous impaction or plugging of airways → air-trapping, hypoventilation, ↑ WOB)
Ventilator malperformance: pooled condensate → ↑ airway pressures or asynchrony with patient (HH)
HME → ineffective low pressure alarm during disconnection

Clinical Goal
Humidified and warmed inspired gases without hazards or complications.

**Adapted from AARC Clinical Practice Guideline: Humidification During Invasive and Noninvasive Mechanical Ventilation, *Respiratory Care*, Vol. 57, #5, 2012.
HH = heated humidity, HME = heat moisture exchanger

Patient-Ventilator Synchrony

Patient synchrony refers to the ventilator's ability to respond to the patient's signal (a trigger, for example). Because the ventilator always has to take some time to respond, there is some asynchrony at baseline.* This section is about ensuring appropriate ventilator response with as minimal a time delay as possible.

Note that while we typically use the term asynchrony and asynchrony interchangeably, there are differences by some authors.

Common Signs of Asynchrony*
- ↑ work of breathing
- Paradoxical breathing (more severe)
- ↑ RR, ↑ HR, ↑ BP
- Graphics are abnormal (double-stacking, missed trigger attempts, etc.). See Graphics Chapter for examples.

The best way to detect presence and cause of asynchrony is for the clinician to spend time at the bedside carefully analyzing graphics, and watching the patient and ventilator simultaneously. Sometimes the best way to optimize synchrony is to use *trial-and-error* by making small changes and watching for response.

Typical Factors Affecting Patient-Ventilator Interaction
Strategies for discovering and addressing each are on the following pages
- Artificial airway
- Auto-PEEP (including I:E ratio)
- Exhalation valve
- Humidity/humidifiers
- Trigger sensitivity
- Mode of ventilation (mode asynchrony)
- Improper flow (flow asynchrony)
- Improper cycle (cycle asynchrony)

* Chatburn R, Mireles-Cabodevila E. 2019 year in review: patient-ventilator synchrony. Respiratory Care; April 2020:65(4)558-572

Artificial Airway
Increases resistance and work of breathing

Common Causes	Potential solutions
ET Tube size too small	• Start with a fairly large ET Tube size (consider 7.5 for women, 8.0 for men) • Consider tube exchange if ↑ WOB and pt has unusually small airway placed • Consider tube compensation (a variable form of pressure support), if available
Patient biting on tube (insert suction catheter to verify patency)	• Consider bite block (caution for skin breakdown) or ET tube holder with integrated bite block design • Carefully consider sedation level
Secretions in Airway (look at graphics, auscultate)	• Suction as needed • Consider bronchoscopy if particularly copious • Consider heated humidity if on an HME and thick secretions

Auto-PEEP (Air trapping)
Increases WOB and asynchrony by flattening the diaphragm, affecting respiratory muscle function, and requiring greater effort to trigger the ventilator.

Common Causes	Potential solutions
Underlying Disease Process (COPD, Asthma, etc.)	• See individual diseases for strategies • Verify expiratory flow returns to baseline (using graphics) • Extend I:E ratio to 1:4 or 1:5
Improperly set I:E ratio	Verify that I:E ratio is adequate, reset TI if necessary

Expiratory (Demand) Valves
Pressure-triggered mechanical demand valves often require large pressure drops to open the valves.

Common Causes	Potential solutions
Valve failing to open appropriately	Use flow-triggered system or Add 5 cmH$_2$O to a demand-flow system
Valve sticking due to aerosolized drugs	For drugs known to cause sticking consider changing expiratory filter regularly, or even using two filters

Humidifiers
Increases resistance and work of breathing

Common Causes	Potential solutions
Bubble-through humidifiers with proximal sensitivity can increase resistance and WOB	Use passover or wick-type humidifiers
HME in patients with secretions that continually collect in HME (increases WOB)	Consider heated humidity instead of HME
Excessive condensate (rain-out) with heated humidity	• Verify correct placement/fit of temperature probes • Verify ambient conditions are optimal (no fan blowing on circuit, etc.) • Ensure circuit positioned to minimize collection of condensate
Thick/difficult to suction secretions	• If HME: consider switching to heated humidity. • If heated humidity: verify adequate heat/humidity.

Management

Trigger Sensitivity

The goal: A patient's inspiratory effort (with minimal duration/intensity) produces a mechanical breath. When this is delayed or fails to occur altogether, it increases the total respiratory effort.

- **Auto-Trigger**: ventilator mistakenly administers a breath (patient didn't intentionally trigger this)
- **Reverse Trigger**: ventilator triggers diaphragmatic muscle contractions in response to passive insufflation of the lungs, resulting in a double breath
- **Missed Trigger**: ventilator fails to administer a breath despite patient making (some) attempt for one

Common Causes	Potential solutions
Leak (Auto-Triggering)	• Verify no leak systematically (disconnect patient from circuit if necessary)
Improper trigger sensitivity or type	• Consider flow trigger when available - this is generally easier to trigger than pressure • Use the most sensitive setting possible without causing auto-triggering • Watch patient's abdomen - as soon as effort is made by patient the ventilator should trigger.
Auto-PEEP	• If changing to flow does not help or is not possible, it may be necessary to increase PEEP to offset auto-PEEP (see pg 7-29)
Flow Sensor Malfunction	• Some ventilators use flow sensors in the patient circuit which may be affected by secretions/condensate/placement (causes auto-triggering) • Ensure flow sensor is operating correctly, attempt to calibrate, replace if necessary
Miscellaneous	Consider impact of: inline nebulizers, HME, ET tube (may delay trigger)

Trigger Sensitivity (continued)

Common Causes	Potential solutions
COPD *(early small airway collapse causes fluctuation in flow, triggering another breath)*	(double triggering) • Decrease flow sensitivity (or switch temporarily to a pressure trigger) • If double-triggering stops, this is likely the cause. • Consider increasing set PEEP (see page 7-29)
Insufficient Inspiratory Time (TI)	• The patient's neural TI may be longer than the set TI • Increase TI 0.1 sec at a time • PSV: decrease inspiratory cycle off to lengthen time
Ineffective Effort	• In some cases, patient effort is inadequate (oversedation, low respiratory drive, hypocarbia) • Consider possible causes, make trigger more sensitive, if possible (and no auto-triggering), consider decreasing sedation
Cardiogenic Oscillations	If too sensitive, particularly with bounding heart rate, the ventilator may auto-trigger. Consider changing to a pressure trigger.
Reverse Triggering	• If the symptoms/triggering worsens with sedation, the cause is likely "reverse triggering" (pt inspiratory effort is delayed, a time lag between the ventilator and the patient's inspiratory effort) • May require NMBA (if affecting clinical status)

Severe (and refractory) asynchrony may occur with some patients due to neural timing issues. Consider the use of a neural-triggered mode (with esophageal probe) if available (NAVA)

Mode Asynchrony (Ventilatory Support)

Mode asynchrony occurs when the ventilator is providing too little or too much support for the patient

Common Causes	Potential solutions
Too much support While higher control modes may rest respiratory muscles, it may also lead to atrophy, and may be uncomfortable for patients with any spontaneous drive	• Avoid using purely control modes of ventilation which "lock" the patient out • Use modes that provide adequate support while allowing for spontaneous triggering • Assess regularly for appropriateness to wean
Inadequate support Leads to fatigue	Differentiate between patient inability and other factors like anxiety which may also cause asynchrony
Unpredictable support May lead to asynchrony - can be thought of as "neural asynchrony" as the brain isn't sure whether the next breath will be ventilator-driven or spontaneous	This may occur with SIMV. Consider using pressure support ventilation with adequate pressure support level (titrate to reasonable RR and V$_T$)

Flow Asynchrony ($\dot{V}_I$ in volume modes)
Inadequate flow leads to an increased WOB

Common Causes	Potential solutions
Inspiratory Airflow Asynchrony Patients with high flow demand may require 60-100 L/min (notable inspiratory effort)	• Assess adequacy of machine flow by observing airway pressure waveform (see Chapter 5). • Adjust $\dot{V}_I$ until airway pressure waveform is restored to normal. • In pressure modes, too long of an inspiratory rise time may lead to ↑WOB • Consider the need to treat pain, dyspnea, delirium/anxiety, or underlying cause of acidosis • Consider trial of pressure mode of ventilation (if on volume) which may be a better physiological match (especially if leaks)

Cycle Asynchrony (TI or Cycle)
Inspiratory Time is set inappropriately usually - patient wants a longer breath, or a shorter breath. Technically this can result in premature cycling, delayed cycling, or false cycling

Common Causes	Potential solutions

Most commonly, the patient attempts to exhale prior to the termination of machine inspiration.
pressure mode:
  T_I is set too long
volume mode:
  flow cycle is prolonged
	Assess and ensure T_I (set or $\dot{V}_I$ result) is adequate (not too short or long) to meet patient's demand
	Flow cycle set too low

Management

Noninvasive Ventilation

Types
- High-Flow Oxygen Therapy 8-2
- CPAP 8-3
- NPPV (BiPAP) 8-4

- Acute Respiratory Failure (Management) 8-8
- Contraindication 8-9
- Interfaces 8-10
- Management Considerations 8-11
- Monitoring for Success 8-12
- Discontinuing 8-12

Terminology
Noninvasive ventilation is one of those areas where terminology, unfortunately, varies widely by source.

- **NIV**: Noninvasive ventilation. Any application of a pressure without use of an artificial invasive airway (ET tube, trach)
- **HFOT**: High-flow oxygen therapy (oxygen given at higher flows than conventional oxygen flows on a flowmeter)
- **HFNC**: High-flow nasal cannula (large bore prongs)
- **CPAP**: Continuous positive airway pressure. Clinically may be noninvasive (prongs, mask) or invasive (by ventilator). Applies constant pressure during inspiration and expiration.
- **NPPV**: Noninvasive positive pressure ventilation. Noninvasive (mask, prongs) ventilation with two pressures (IPAP and EPAP). Other common names: BiPAP (brand name), Bilevel positive airway pressure
- **IPAP**: Inspiratory Positive Airway Pressure: high pressure setting during NPPV
- **EPAP**: Expiratory Positive Airway Pressure: low pressure setting during NPPV

High-Flow Oxygen Therapy (HFOT)
High-Flow Nasal Cannula (HFNC)

Effects
- High flowrate washes out CO_2 from anatomic deadspace (does not provide a tidal volume)
- May help decrease WOB
- PEEP-like effect from mix of added flow to inspiration, then resistance during exhalation. While not easily measurable, it is thought to be linear (higher flowrate = higher PEEP-like effect)

Specific Indications*
- Mild-to-moderate acute hypoxemic respiratory failure
- Mild-to-moderate acute hypercapnic respiratory failure (especially if NIV mask intolerance): does not enhance tidal volume, but helps wash out CO_2.
- Post-extubation bridge therapy (may help prevent reintubation)
- Patients who have a Do-Not-Intubate (DNI) with respiratory distress
- Acute heart failure with hypoxemia and dyspnea
- When intubating, consider pre-oxygenating with HFNC (assuming ventilatory drive), keep in place during intubation attempts. Initiating HFNC for this purpose is controversial.

Hazards
- Aspiration risk (use caution with eating/drinking with high flow)
- Skin breakdown (monitor closely, consider use of skin barrier devices at points of contact)

Initiation
- Large bore soft nasal cannula is utilized. Proper fit is usually "snug but not tight" (some leak is desirable to minimize the risk of skin breakdown) (a sizing tool is often available from the manufacturer)
- Initiate at a lower flow/higher FiO_2. Spend time with patient to ensure comfort and compliance. Then, titrate flow higher and wean FiO_2 until meeting oxygenation target.

*Nishimura M. High-flow nasal cannula oxygen therapy in adults: physiological benefits, indication, clinical benefits, and adverse effects. Respiratory Care; April 2016:61(4)529-541

HFNC Suggested Settings

Flow	20-60 L/min
	Initiate at lower flow until patient is comfortable Then, titrate per clinical effect ($FiO_2 < 0.50$) and patient tolerance Flow may create a PEEP-like effect (debated)
FiO_2	0.21 to 1.0
	For acute respiratory failure start high, then wean per goals
Humidity	Use heated humidity (some clinicians perform a very short trial without humidity to verify patient tolerance to therapy)

Management and Weaning/Discontinuation

- Assess frequently for tolerance, clinical goals, and skin integrity
- Once clinical goals met ($FiO_2 < 0.50$, WOB at baseline), consider for weaning unless underlying cause has not begun to reverse
- Reduce flow in increments of 5-10 L/min, then monitor patient closely. If worsening vital signs, WOB, increase flow and discontinue wean.
- Once at ~20 L/min, consider transitioning to convention oxygen device (nasal cannula)

Noninvasive Continuous Positive Airway Pressure (CPAP)
For CPAP applied invasively, see Modes Chapter

- Provides a constant pressure throughout inspiration and expiration
- During inspiration provides support
- During expiration provides expiratory resistance

Specific Indications
- Hypoxemic respiratory failure when due to atelectasis or airway collapse
- Acute cardiogenic pulmonary edema (CHF)

Initiation
- Ensure proper size and fit of mask interface (see page 8-10)
- Ensure adequate time is spent with the patient to reduce anxiety, ensure optimization of fit/settings, and assess overall tolerance. It may benefit to allow patient to hold mask on own face without straps initially.

Suggested Settings

CPAP	5-20 cmH$_2$O pressures > 20 cmH$_2$O may increase risk of gastric insufflation
F$_IO_2$	0.21-1.0
Humidity	Use heated humidity

Management
- Increase CPAP by increments until F$_IO_2$ can be weaned below 0.50
- Once clinically stable, consider the ability to wean. Wean CPAP in increments of 1-2 cmH$_2$O until around 5 cmH$_2$O. Then, discontinue and place on conventional oxygen therapy.

Noninvasive Positive Pressure Ventilation (NPPV)
While a brand name, this is often referred to as BiPAP at the bedside.

- Provides two pressures: a high pressure (IPAP) and a low pressure (EPAP)
- EPAP is similar to PEEP (primarily an oxygenation variable)
- IPAP-EPAP (ΔP) determines support (primarily a ventilation variable)

Specific Indications
- Hypercapnic respiratory failure with or without hypoxemic respiratory failure (COPD exacerbation, etc.)
- Hypoxemic respiratory failure when an increased work of breathing is observed

Initiation
- Ensure proper size and fit of mask interface (see page 8-10)
- Ensure adequate time is spent with the patient to reduce anxiety, ensure optimization of fit/settings, and assess overall tolerance. It may benefit to allow patient to hold mask on own face without straps initially.

IPAP	inspiratory positive airway pressure	ΔP = IPAP - EPAP • Increasing or decreasing ΔP will affect ventilation (similar to V_T) • Increasing or decreasing EPAP will affect oxygenation (similar to PEEP)
EPAP	expiratory positive airway pressure	

Noninvasive

Suggested Settings

IPAP	10-20 cmH$_2$O
	• Ensure 5+ above EPAP at all times to allow for adequate ventilation/support
	• IPAP is only titrated to manipulate the dP (increasing ΔP will increase V$_T$; decreasing ΔP will decrease V$_T$)
	• IPAP of > 20 may increase risk of gastric insufflation (air in stomach)
EPAP	5-19 cmH$_2$O
	• Titrate based on oxygenation (similar to PEEP)
F$_I$O$_2$	0.21-1.0
Humidity	Use heated humidity

Management

- Oxygenation
  - Increase EPAP (and IPAP by the same) incrementally until F$_I$O$_2$ is weaned to < 0.50 (or until at 20 cmH$_2$O)
- Ventilation
  - Manipulate the ΔP (IPAP - EPAP), usually by increasing IPAP (while decreasing EPAP will also widen the ΔP, this may have a detrimental effect on oxygenation goals)
  - In general, increasing ΔP will increase V$_T$. Decreasing ΔP will decrease V$_T$.
  - Note that if making changes to both oxygenation and ventilation simultaneously, the IPAP and ΔP will need to be titrated together

Examples with an initial setting of 10/5 cmH$_2$O

Baseline example settings:	10/5 IPAP 10 EPAP 5 ΔP (IPAP - EPAP) = 5
Improve oxygenation	12/7 (from baseline above) ↑ IPAP to 12 ↑ EPAP to 7 (↑ Oxygenation) maintain ΔP (IPAP - EPAP) = 5
Increase ventilation	12/5 (from baseline above) ↑ IPAP to 12 maintain EPAP at 5 ↑ ΔP (IPAP - EPAP) = 7 (↑ V$_T$)
Improve both oxygenation and ventilation	14/7 (from baseline above) ↑ IPAP to 14 ↑ EPAP to 7 (↑ Oxygenation) ↑ ΔP (IPAP - EPAP) = 7 (↑ V$_T$)

Noninvasive Management
(Acute Respiratory Failure)

Verify indications for noninvasive management*:
- Acute hypoxemia (SpO$_2$ < 88-90% with FIO$_2$ > 0.60) and/or
- Acute hypercapnic failure:
  - Worsening dyspnea (usually severe)
  - Sustained tachypnea (> 25 breaths/min)
  - Increased WOB (accessory muscles, abdominal paradox)
  - pH < 7.35 with PaCO$_2$ increased from baseline

Are there Contraindications?
(see next page) — Yes → **Intubate** Consider need to intubate and initiate invasive ventilation

↓ No

Initiate carefully monitored trial (30-60 minutes) of NIV:
- HFNC or CPAP if hypoxemic
- NPPV if hypercapnic

Titrate settings, adjust interface per clinical effect and patient tolerance

Reasonable Improvement?
(see next page) — No →

↓ Yes

Maintain settings
(wean FIO$_2$ towards baseline, as able)

→ No

Weaning (liberated within 24-hours?)
Give initial short break (10-15 min), assess carefully.
Increase time off NIV each break.

*See Disease Chapter for specific indications by disease/disorder

Contraindications to Providing NIV

Absolute (avoid use)
- Apnea
- Cardiopulmonary arrest
- Facial burns
- Facial or cranial trauma
- Fixed upper airway obstruction
- Hemodynamic instability/arrhythmias
- Inability to protect airway/vomiting (risk of aspiration)
- Need for immediate intubation and airway protection
- Severe epistaxis
- Severe respiratory acidosis (pH < 7.20)
- Upper gastrointestinal (GI) bleeding

Relative (consider in context of patient assessment)
- Anxiety/claustrophobia
- Inability to tolerate therapy/interface (dementia, etc.)
- Bowel obstruction
- Copious secretions
- Inability to clear secretions
- Severe illness (high APACHE score)

Assessment of Improvement

Unless being used for palliative care, NIV should be viewed as a trial. Evidence of stabilization/improvement should occur within a reasonable period. If either deterioration or lack of improvement, consider the need for invasive ventilation.

Verify Patient Status	• Adequate mental status • Tolerance of therapy and interface
Assessment	↓ RR, ↓ BP, ↓ HR, ↓ WOB, ↓ dyspnea, breath sounds improving/stable
Stable/improved Oxygenation	• Ability to decrease FiO_2 (goal is < 50%), with • Oxygenation (SpO_2, PaO_2, P/F ratio, S/F ratio) meeting minimal goals (SpO_2 > 92%, for example)
Stable/improved ventilation	Improved ventilation ($PaCO_2$, $ETCO_2$, V_T, RR) (or stable if baseline was acceptable)

Patient Interfaces: Masks
Initiation and Assessment

A mask is most common for acute care settings, although there are technically several designs:
- Nasal mask (covers just nares, straps onto head)
- Face mask (covers mouth and nose) sitting on upper chin and bridge of nose. Most common in acute care.
- Full face mask (covers full face), intended for patients with claustrophobia or certain traumas

Fitting
Care must be given to appropriately sizing mask, ensuring straps are snug but not tight, and that the patient is adequately calm (excessive movement or anxiety can interrupt fit)

Fit too tight	*Usually caused when strapped on tightly to eliminate leak and/or mask is too small* • Increases risk of skin breakdown • Decreases patient comfort/compliance
Fit well	*Fit is snug but not tight* • Slight leak is normal, desired • Leak is compensated by the equipment (see manufacturer literature for details on max leak allowable)
Fit too loose	*Leak around mask is beyond that which the equipment can compensate for, may be due to being strapped incorrectly, too loosely, or incorrectly sized mask* • Decreased pressure delivery (will be below what is set) • Decreases patient comfort/compliance

Assessment
Assess frequently for:
- Signs of skin breakdown, esp. at bridge of nose (use a skin barrier, ensure appropriate, not overly tight, fit)
- Amount of leak around edges of mask (some leak is desirable)
- Condition of mask (secretions, etc.)

Management Considerations

Goals of NPPV in Acute Respiratory Failure	• Avoid intubation and its complications • Improve or stabilize gas exchange • Reduce work of breathing • Relieve dyspnea
Clinical benefits of NPPV in Acute Respiratory Failure	• May decrease need for sedation • Preserves airway defenses/speech/swallowing • Avoids risk of ventilator-associated events (VAP, etc.) • May reduce the need for intubation with associated risk of morbidity, mortality • May shorten the length of stay
Factors that may Predict Success	• Ability to control secretions • Mask leak appropriately managed • Appropriate level of consciousness • Improvement in pH, $PaCO_2$, respiratory rate, and accessory muscle use after 1 hour of NPPV
Factors that may Predict Failure	• Deterioration or lack of improvement in clinical status • Worsening level of consciousness • Development of complications, new symptoms • Patient intolerance of interface • Patient intolerance of settings needed to stabilize (flow too high)
Complications	• Aspiration • Hypotension • Pneumothorax • Uncontrolled leaks that affect ability of equipment to deliver pressure • Dry upper airway • Gastric distension • Discomfort/intolerance • Skin integrity issues (breakdown)

Monitoring for NIV Success

- Once NIV is initiated, close observation is required to assess success or failure

- Improvement should occur within 1-2 hours (consider this a trial period).
  Assess for the following:
  - Improved acid-base status (pH improves with $PaCO_2$ improving towards baseline normal)
  - Patient tolerance/comfort (decreased RR, improved WOB, evidence of synchronization with NIV)
  - Stable overall clinical status (mental status, cardiovascular status, vital signs including SpO_2 and $ETCO_2$)
- Based on improvement/stabilization and clinical judgment, an additional period of optimizing settings may be indicated (adjusting parameters, interface, humidity, etc.), but avoid delays to intubate when patient is clinically deteriorating

Considerations for Discontinuing NIV (NIV Failure)
Evidence suggests as many as 1/3 of patients fail an initial NIV trial. In most cases, this implies the need to intubate and initiate invasive ventilation.

- Worsening or unimproving oxygenation (SpO_2, PaO_2, P/F ratio)
- Worsening or unimproving ventilation ($ETCO_2$, $PaCO_2$)
- Worsening vital signs (hypotension, tachypnea, tachycardia)
- Intolerance of interface (pulling off, refusing, etc.)
- Intolerance of necessary parameters
- Evidence of barotrauma
- Hemodynamic instability
- Inability to clear secretions (evidence or risk of aspiration)
- Worsening agitation or combativeness
- Decreasing mental status
- Worsening encephalopathy

9 Diseases/Disorders

ARDS	9-2
Asthma	9-11
Bariatrics	9-16
Bronchopleural Fistula	9-18
Burns (Thermal, Smoke Inhalation)	9-20
Cardiac, Acute (MI, CHF)	9-22
Cardiac, Postoperative	9-24
COPD Exacerbations	9-25
COVID (see Viral Pulmonary Disorders)	
Drug Overdose	9-29
Guillain-Barre Syndrome (see Neuromuscular)	
Lung Abscess (see Unilateral Disorders)	
Lung Transplantation (see Unilateral Disorders)	
Myasthenia Gravis (see Neuromuscular)	
Neuromuscular Disorders	9-31
Pneumonia (see Unilateral Disorders)	
Poisoning (see Drug Overdose)	
Postoperative Care	9-33
Restrictive Disorders	9-34
Trauma (Chest)	9.35
Trauma (Head)	9-38
Unilateral Disorders	9-42
Independent Lung Ventilation	9-43
Viral Pulmonary Disorders	9-44

DISEASES

Notes
- The primary goals of this chapter are to provide noninvasive (when appropriate) and invasive settings and management strategies for each disease.
- While patients with diseases/disorders may follow a pattern of signs and symptoms, each person's care should be individualized, especially with the large percentage of patients with multiple comorbidities.

Diseases/Disorders

Acute Respiratory Distress Syndrome (ARDS)

An acute, diffuse inflammatory lung injury resulting in diminished functional residual capacity, severe shunting, alveolar transudates, atelectasis, decreased compliance, and refractory hypoxemia.

Pathophysiology
Three phases with some overlap and variation between them:
- **Phase 1: Exudative (first 7-10 days)**
  Intense inflammatory response, resulting in:
  - Alveolar and endothelial damage
  - Increased vascular permeability = pulmonary edema
  - Type II cell hyperplasia
  - Hyaline membrane formation

- **Phase 2 Proliferative (10+ days)**
  Repair and regeneration occur, resulting in:
  - Pulmonary edema resolves
  - Type II cells regenerate, replacing surfactant loss
  - Some level of fibrosis (collagen deposits, interstitial infiltration)

- **Phase 3: Fibrotic Phase**
  Varies, not apparent in all patients, severity varies widely:
  - Fibrosis
  - Damage/remodeling of lung structures

Etiology
There are many possible causes of ARDS, but some of the most common include:
- **Sepsis (most common)**
- Aspiration (~1/3 of pts who aspirate in hospital develop ARDS)
- Cardiopulmonary bypass (post-perfusion injury)
- Lung transplantation
- Pancreatitis
- Pneumonia: Community-acquired and Healthcare-acquired
- Transfusions (massive)
- Trauma (severe, including lung contusions, fat emboli, tissue injury, drowning, burns)

Diagnosis
There are 4 clinical criteria for diagnosis (Berlin definition):
1. **Acute Onset of Respiratory Distress**
   Must be within 7 days of a defined event (sepsis, trauma, pneumonia, etc.). Most cases occur within 72 hours.

2. **Hypoxemia:**

Severity of ARDS	PaO$_2$/FIO$_2$ ratio (P/F) (on PEEP ≥ 5 cmH$_2$O)
Mild	200 - 300
Moderate	100 - 200
Severe	< 100

3. **Bilateral consolidation on CXR or CT scan**
   Bilateral infiltrates - diffuse or not (pulmonary edema)

4. **Ruled out cardiac failure and fluid overload**
   Determined either by PCWP < 18 cmH$_2$O (noncardiogenic), or by clinical examination (because PA catheters are less common, examination techniques, such as echocardiography, are acceptable)

Clinical Manifestations
Significant hypoxemia in initial phase, usually refractory. May note a steady increase in need for supplemental O$_2$ (with minimal to no improvement in PaO$_2$). Symptoms often worsen to respiratory failure.

Physical Exam	Increasing respiratory distress: tachypnea, tachycardia, ↑ work of breathing, dyspnea, dull percussion	
Auscultation	Coarse crackles (pulmonary edema) Bronchial breath sounds (consolidation)	
ABGs	Early	Respiratory alkalosis* with hypoxemia
	Later	Respiratory acidosis* with severe hypoxemia
	* If underlying cause of ARDS is metabolic, there will be a metabolic component to ABG	

Diseases/Disorders

Imaging	Often "white out" of lungs (ground glass appearance): bilateral infiltrates (often diffuse), air bronchograms
Hemodynamics	PCWP Normal or ↓ CVP ↑ Hemodynamics may also be determined by underlying cause (such as septic shock)
Pulmonary Dynamics	Decreased compliance Increased PIP on ventilator V/Q mismatch

ARDS Ventilator Management

The goal of treatment with ARDS is largely protective (protect the lungs from as much damage as possible), supportive (support failing systems), and treatment-based (treat underlying cause):

Lung Protection	Lung protective ventilator strategies (maintaining plateau pressures < 30 or driving pressure < 15 using low VT strategy, allowing permissive hypercapnia)
Supportive	**Support failing systems:** **Oxygenation** (refractory hypoxemia is likely): Optimize O_2: use of PEEP (vs FIO_2) or other recruitment strategies (mode, etc.), patient positioning - proning (improves V/Q), Decrease O_2 consumption: ensure synchrony on ventilator (mode, settings, sedation), treat pain and fever, etc. **Hemodynamics**: monitor closely (CVP, A-Line), maintain mean arterial pressure > 60 to ensure adequate perfusion
Treatment	Treat underlying causes when possible (see etiologies for common causes)

Noninvasive Management
Noninvasive care is appropriate for some patients, but many clinicians use a low threshold of failure (at first sign of failure, consider intubation)

Consider a trial of noninvasive if patient meets criteria:
- Mild ARDS (see pg 9-3)
- Hemodynamically stable
- Able to tolerate patient interface (prongs, mask)
- Meets normal criteria for noninvasive therapy (see pg 8-9)

Assess patient carefully during the trial. If any deterioration, consider need for invasive ventilation.

Invasive Management
Suggested settings on following page

- Consider more aggressive approach to timing of intubation (do not delay until full respiratory failure)
- Keep in mind goals (see previous page): ultimate goal is to protect the lungs while maintaining life (minimum thresholds for oxygenation and ventilation)
- While Pplat has been conventionally followed, consider optimizing settings using driving pressure (higher PEEP with lower Pplat). See page 2-14.
- If invasive ventilation strategies fail, consider alternatives:
  - APRV (TCAV)
  - Inhaled pulmonary vasodilators (improve oxygenation, not mortality)
  - HFOV (don't use routinely, *ATS 2017*)
  - ECMO (mixed evidence, *ATS 2017*)

Diseases/Disorders

ARDS Ventilator Settings

Mode	Limited evidence to support one mode over another, but ensure a consistent delivery of low V_T (lung protective approach)
V_T	**6-8 mL/kg IBW** (check Pplat, target V_T to keep ≤ 30 cmH$_2$O, as low as 4 mL/kg may be necessary)
f	**12+/min** (titrate to maintain minimum pH via PaCO$_2$) Note: It's common to increase *f* in order to maintain low tidal volumes. Ensure time for exhalation to baseline to avoid complications of auto-PEEP.
T$_I$	**0.8 - 1.2 sec** *Note*: lengthen T$_I$ to improve oxygenation only after V_T, *f* and PEEP have been optimized. ↑ in 0.1 sec increments to achieve oxygenation target (rather than a specific I:E ratio)
PEEP	**5+ cmH$_2$O** increase incrementally until F$_I$O$_2$ < 60 torr (without causing overdistension)
F$_I$O$_2$	As needed to achieve PaO$_2$ target (~ 60 torr)
Other	• Ensure alarms alert to a clinical increase in VT • Set pressure limits (high pressure alarm) when mode allows for it • See APRV (TCAV) page 3-20

ARDS Management Strategies

All management is aimed at preventing lung injury while maintaining minimally adequate oxygenation and ventilation.

Ventilation
- Allow for permissive hypercapnia (see ABGs, below)
- V_T to as low as 4 mL/kg when P_{alv} > 30 cmH$_2$O
- Increase f to maintain minimum PCO$_2$ (avoid auto-PEEP)
- Pplat > 30 cmH$_2$O may be acceptable in conditions with poor chest wall compliance (obesity, etc.)

Oxygenation
- In general, goal is to maintain minimal oxygenation goal using as little supplemental oxygen as possible (F$_I$O$_2$ < 0.5 if possible)
- Use ARDSnet PEEP strategies (see page 9-8), generally higher than normal PEEP (but avoid over distension)
- Consider use of recruitment (proning for 12-16 hrs, recruitment maneuvers) in short trial (abandon if no improvement)

Arterial Blood Gas Targets

PaO$_2$: Mild ARDS ≥ 70 mmHg **pH:** > 7.15
Moderate ARDS ≥ 60 mmHg **PaCO$_2$:**
Severe ARDS ≥ 55 mmHg (Intentional Hypercapnia)

Permissive hypercapnia (PaCO$_2$ < 100 mmHg) is permissible to limit Pplat ≤ 30 cmH$_2$O. It is usually a necessity once auto-PEEP develops (unless contraindicated or ↑ ICP)

Weaning/Liberation
- Stabilize patient. Once oxygenation shows improvement, consider ability to wean.
- No one weaning attempt has been proven superior over any other. See ARDSnet guidelines in pages following for more details.

Diseases/Disorders

ARDSnet PROTOCOL Information

See ardsnet.org for complete details. Note that evidence support varies.

FiO₂/PEEP Tables*

Low PEEP Approach		High PEEP Approach	
FiO₂	PEEP	FiO₂	PEEP
0.3	5	0.3	12
0.4	5	0.3	14
0.4	8	0.4	14
0.5	8	0.4	16
0.5	10	0.5	16
0.6	10	0.5	18
0.7	10	0.5-0.8	20
0.7	12	0.8	22
0.7	14	0.9	22
0.8	14	1.0	22-24
0.9	14		
0.9	16		
0.9	18		
1.0	18		
1.0	20-24		
1.0	26-34*		

*NHLBI ARDS Clinical Trials Network. Higher versus lower positive end-expiratory pressures in patients with the acute respiratory distress syndrome. **N Engl J Med** 351: 327-336, 2004

Protocol Ranges: PaO₂ 55-80 mmHg, SpO₂ 88-95%
Note: Mild hypoxemia is preferred over high levels of FiO₂ and PEEP. Promptly ↓ FiO₂ and PEEP levels when upper levels are reached.

In the presence of severe hypoxemia or severe acidosis:
Pplat limit of 30 cmH₂O may be temporarily suspended.

When severe patient-ventilator asynchrony occurs:
V$_T$ may be ↑ to 7 - 8 mL/kg as long as Pplat ≤ 30 cmH₂O.
Set *f* to 6 - 35 breaths/min to maintain pH 7.30-7.45.

ARDSNET Protocol Adjustments

Condition	Strategy
P_{plat} > 30 cmH$_2$O	↓ V$_T$ by 1 mL/kg PBW every 2-3 hr, no less than 4 mL/kg PBW ↑ f to maintain $\dot{V}_E$
Pplat < 25 cmH$_2$O and V$_T$ < 6 mL/kg	↑ V$_T$ to 6 mL/kg PBW and ↓ f to maintain $\dot{V}_E$
Mild acidosis: pH 7.15-7.30	↑ f to 35 breaths/min or until pH ≥ 7.30 with PaCO$_2$ ≥ 25 mmHg. If pH remains < 7.30 and PaCO$_2$ < 25 mmHg, consider treatment with NaHCO$_3$.
Severe acidosis: pH < 7.15	↑ f to 35 breaths/min and consider treatment of pH with NaHCO$_3$. If pH remains < 7.15, ↑ V$_T$ by 1 mL/kg until pH > 7.15. Pplat > 30 cmH$_2$O is acceptable Upper limits of V$_T$ and Pplat are suspended until pH = 7.20.
Severe hypoxemia: PaO$_2$ < 55 mmHg (SpO$_2$ < 88%) on FiO$_2$ 1.0 and PEEP 24 cmH$_2$O	Upper limits of V$_T$ and Pplat are suspended during PEEP trial between 26 and 34 cmH$_2$O. I:E is set at 1:1.
Severe patient-ventilator asynchrony: The failure of the ventilator to pressurize the circuit above PEEP during inspiration, or double-triggering the ventilator during inspiration (> 3/min).	↑ f and ↓ I:E to ↑ $\dot{V}_I$ Maximize trigger sensitivity If available on VV, use decelerating flow pattern to ↑ $\dot{V}_I$. If above measures ineffective and Pplat < 30 cmH$_2$O, ↑ V$_T$ by 1 mL/kg up to 8 mL.

Monitor Hemodynamic Status Closely: response to low V$_T$ ventilation (including hypercapnia, respiratory acidosis, sedation, low V$_T$, high PEEP, patient's underlying disease, etc.) is complex

Weaning evaluation begins when:
- Stable Oxygenation on FiO_2 0.4 and PEEP ≤ 8
- Systolic BP ≥ 90 mmHg without vasopressors
- No neuromuscular blockade
- Patient exhibiting inspiratory efforts

Weaning Assessment
5 min CPAP trial
(FiO_2 0.5 with CPAP 5)

f ≤ 35 breaths/min — no signs of intolerance

Pressure Support Trial
- FiO_2 0.5
- PS determined by f at end of CPAP trial

f > 35 breaths/min and/or intolerance

Return to A/C until next day
If f >35 is due to anxiety, adjust sedation and may attempt a second CPAP trial within 4 hrs.

f = 26-35
PS = 20 above PEEP
PEEP = 5
- ↓ PS by 5 every 1-3 hr when f ≤ 35 (or every 5 min when f < 25)
- ↑ PS by 5 when f > 35
- If PS level ≥15 by 1900, or if f >35 on PS 20, return to A/C
- Retry PS weaning between 0600 and 1000 next day

f < 25
PS = 5 above PEEP
PEEP = 5
- After 2h of PS=5, f≤35 and no signs of intolerance, go to CPAP trial
- ↑ PS by 5 when f > 35
- If PS level ≤ 10 at 1900, maintain PS overnight

After 2h-trial of CPAP 5:
- f ≤ 35
- PaO_2 ≥ 60 (or SpO_2 ≥ 90%) with pH ≥ 7.30
- V_T ≥ 4 mL/kg
- Absence of intolerance

Unassisted Breathing
Extubation w/ Supp O_2
T-Piece
Trach-Collar
CPAP 5 with no PS or IMV

Adapted from Kallet R, Corral W, Silverman H, Luce J. Implementation of a low tidal volume ventilation protocol for patients with acute lung injury or acute respiratory distress syndrome. *Resp Care* 2001;46(10):1024-1037

Asthma

A disease of chronic airway inflammation with evidence of variable expiratory airflow limitation. Patients experience variable respiratory symptoms (wheeze, shortness of breath, chest tightness, and/or cough) consistent with airways that overrespond (hyperresponsiveness) to stimuli (allergens, etc.) by narrowing and producing mucus.

Pathophysiology

- **Inflammation of the airways**
  An overreaction to normal stimuli/allergens:
  - Antibodies develop after exposure to a stimulus
  - These stimuli "trigger" an overresponse
  - Mast cells, once triggered, degranulate and produce an inflammatory response

- **Bronchial hyperresponsiveness**
  Smooth muscles contract in an overreaction to normal stimuli

- **Airway remodeling**
  Permanent changes to the structure of the airways that result in irreversible obstruction in at least some patients
  - Increase in goblet cells (increasing mucus production)
  - Thickening of the bronchial walls
  - Change in smooth muscle function/structure resulting in air-trapping (dynamic hyperinflation)

Acid-Base
Early: Acute respiratory alkalosis with hypoxemia
Late: Acute respiratory acidosis with severe hypoxemia

A normal ABG with hypoxemia and respiratory distress indicates impending respiratory arrest

Indications for Ventilator Support
- Acute respiratory failure*
- Hyper-expansion on CXR
- Diminished air flow on auscultation (or absent)
- Exhaustion (↑ or ↓ RR and decreased mental status)
- Life-threatening dysrhythmias
- Respiratory/Cardiac Arrest
- Severe refractory hypoxemia

Asthma Noninvasive Management
Use of NPPV is controversial but may support a patient's ventilatory needs for a short trial (to allow time for steroids and bronchodilators to become effective)

Limitations of NPPV:
- Increases risk of aspiration
- May cause heightened sense of air hunger
- High risk of auto-PEEP

Initial Settings:
When $FIO_2 < 0.70$ / $PaCO_2 < 50$ mmHg:

CPAP	Start at 5 cmH₂O and titrate for SpO_2
FIO_2	1.0, then wean as clinically indicated

When $FIO_2 > 0.70$ / $PaCO_2 > 50$ mmHg

NPPV	start at IPAP 8-10 / EPAP 3-5 Titrate up to 10-12 / 5-7 Maintain ΔP (IPAP - EPAP) of at least 5 cmH₂O
FIO_2	1.0, then wean as clinically indicated

Failure to improve after a short trial may be an indication for intubation

Asthma Invasive Management

Do not delay intubation once determined to be necessary:
- Lack of improvement or increased WOB on NPPV
- Persistent hypercapnia ($PaCO_2$ > 50 mmHg)
- Refractory hypoxemia (FIO_2 > 0.60)
- Altered mental status

Caution: manipulation of the airway may cause increased obstruction due to exaggerated bronchial responsiveness

Suggested Ventilator Settings

Mode	• No specific mode (optimize settings instead)
V_T	Starting V_T 6-8 mL/kg IBW Decrease V_T to keep PIP < 40 and Pplat < 30
f	Lower Rates (8-12 breaths/min) Rationale: Prevent auto-PEEP
T_I	0.75 - 1.2 sec Verify T_E is adequate for exhalation (use flow scalar or measure auto-PEEP) High $\dot{V}_I$ (80 - 100 L/min) I:E of 1:3 to 1:5
FIO_2	Wean for SpO_2 > 90-92%
PEEP	5-8 cmH_2O, then titrate as needed (60-80% of auto-PEEP, allows for distal airway emptying)

- Monitor closely for auto-PEEP
- Asynchrony with the vent is common. Optimize settings (trigger, etc.), then consider need for increased sedation and possibly NMBAs.

National Asthma Education Guidelines*

Signs of Impending Respiratory Failure:
  Altered mental state
  Worsening fatigue
  $PaCO_2 \geq 42$

Intubation: DO NOT DELAY ONCE DEEMED NECESSARY (see Near-Fatal Asthma below for intubation indications and procedure.)
Heliox (Heliox-driven Albuterol treatments) or magnesium sulfate may be considered to avoid intubation.

Mechanical Ventilation - Initial Settings

V_T	6 - 10 mL/kg (volume modes)
	($\downarrow V_T$ to keep PIP < 35 cmH$_2$O)
PV:	keep PIP ≤ 30 - 35 cmH$_2$O
f	12 – 25 breaths/min
PEEP	4 - 10 cmH$_2$O
F_iO_2	1.0
T_I	Keep short enough to ensure expiration ends before next inspiration.

Clinical Notes: Immediately assess for chest rise, BS, airflow, and T_E. Monitor for auto-PEEP and barotrauma. Monitor with end-tidal CO$_2$
Permissive hypercapnia is the recommended strategy, but it is not uniformly successful. Minimize high airway pressures and barotrauma.

*Adapted from the *Guidelines for the Diagnosis and Management of Asthma, the National Asthma Education Program's Expert Panel: Report 2, 1998, and EPR-3, 2007*; National Heart Lung, and Blood Institute; National Institutes of Health, Bethesda, MD.

Diseases/Disorders

Asthma Strategies for Severe Exacerbations

Hypotension After Intubating
Check for tension pneumothorax:
- 1-unilateral chest expansion; 2-tracheal shift; 3-subcutaneous emphysema (crepitus)
- Decompression – insert 16 gauge needle into 2nd IC space, mid-clavicular line. Insert chest tube if air is emitted.

Check and treat auto-PEEP (commonly causes hypotension)
- Stop ventilation for < 1 min to allow auto-PEEP to dissipate.
- Decrease inhalation time (increasing exhalation indirectly)
- Decrease f by 2 breaths/min at a time
- Decrease V$_T$ down to 3-5 mL/kg IBW
- Observe oxygenation.

Bronchoconstriction
- Intubation and ventilation can further exacerbate
- Assess breath sounds, acid-base, Raw (PIP - Pplat)
- Consider aggressive use of SABAs (continuous, high-dose)
- Consider continued systemic corticosteroids
- Suction as needed for excessive secretions (Consider BAL, but bronchoconstriction may temporarily worsen)
- Consider heliox (if vent is calibrated for it)
- ECMO may benefit if refractory acidosis

If airway is difficult to ventilate, perform the following, in order, until ventilation is adequate*:
1. Ensure optimized patient-ventilator interaction
2. Asses ET tube for patency.
3. Ensure adequate V$_T$: ↑ T$_E$, ↓T$_I$ and ↑ PIP
4. Decrease rate to 6-8/min (to ↓ auto-PEEP to ≤ 15 cmH$_2$O)
5. Decrease V$_T$ to 3-5 mL/kg (to ↓ auto-PEEP to ≤ 15 cmH$_2$O
6. Increase flow to > 60 L/min

---

*Brief Synopsis of the Guidelines 2000 for Cardiopulmonary Resuscitation and Emergency Cardiovascular Care: International Consensus on Science. AHA and the International Liaison Committee of Resuscitation, Circulation, 2000; 102 (Suppl I): I-1-384, and 2005 Update; Circulation, 2005, Vol 112, No. 24; Circulation, 2010

Diseases/Disorders

Bariatrics (Obesity)

Obese patients have altered metabolism and pulmonary mechanics which impact on critical care management. The degree to which this occurs is usually dependent on the severity of obesity (BMI) and activity level.

Pathophysiology
- Airway collapse (upper, lower) leads to air trapping, obstruction, increased work of breathing
- Atelectasis (shunting)
- Decreased expiratory reserve volume (ERV, including FRC and IRV)
- Increased metabolic rate (↑ O_2 consumption and CO_2 production)
- Obesity hypoventilation syndrome at baseline

Noninvasive Strategies
NIV, either CPAP (OSA) or NPPV (OSA, OHS) may be required at baseline for some of these patients. Increasing use (duration, non-typical times like daytime use vs. night use) of these during an acute hospitalization is logical (with analgesia, anesthesia, etc.), and baseline settings may need to be titrated acutely

CPAP	Typically 15-25 cmH_2O for oxygenation
NPPV	NPPV when respiratory insufficiency (with or without oxygenation issue)
FiO_2	O_2 reserves may be lower, titrate to clinical goals

- Ensure appropriate mask fit (leaks are more common, but avoid strapping too tightly due to risk of skin breakdown). Nasal interfaces may be worth initial trial (prongs, mask)
- For use with respiratory distress, improvement should be noted within a reasonable period. If none, or worsening, intubation may be necessary.

Obesity Invasive Management

Uncommon to intubate solely based on obesity, but usually there is an underlying acute process (surgery, trauma, illness, etc.)

Suggested Ventilator Settings

V_T	Starting V_T 6-8 mL/kg IBW It is critical to measure the patient's height and base V_T or V_T target on height, not body weight. Avoid adding V_T to compensate for weight (consider PEEP instead)
f	Higher Rates (15+ breaths/min) due to increased metabolic rates
T_I	0.75 - 1.2 sec
F_IO_2	Wean for SpO_2 > 90-92%
PEEP	Higher PEEP to offset chest wall, abdominal pressures (as high as 10-20 cmH_2O) (assess hemodynamics to ensure no over-distension)

- Plateau pressures should be maintained < 35 cmH_2O with increased PEEP. Esophageal manometry is helpful in determining chest wall and abdominal pressures (versus actual lung compliance)

Weaning/Discontinuation

- Consider spontaneous breathing trial with same level of PEEP needed for CPAP (or EPAP from NPPV)

Diseases/Disorders

Bronchopleural Fistula (B-P Fistula)

A pathway exists between the bronchus (main stem, lobar, or segmental) and the pleural space, which can be caused by trauma, surgery, invasive procedures, or certain diseases (necrotizing pneumonia, etc.)

Type of Ventilation
- A ventilator capable of delivering high $\dot{V}_I$ and large V_T may be required when a large air leak is present
- Pressure modes may help control peak alveolar pressures
- Low-rate SIMV or PSV may help minimize the number of full ventilator-given breaths
- Avoid PSV IF B-P fistula leak is greater than the flow level required to terminate inspiration as the ventilator will not cycle from I to E

Note: Non-conventional approaches include ILV and HFV. Neither have been shown to improve outcome.

Mode	Pressure ventilation may control peak alveolar pressures
V_T	4-8 mL/kg IBW
f	10-30 breaths/min (depends on underlying process)
Flow ($\dot{V}_I$)	70 - 100 L/min with decelerating pattern
PEEP	0 - 10 cmH$_2$O (minimize when possible)

Diseases/Disorders

Indication for Mechanical Ventilation
B-P fistula in itself is not an indication for ventilation. Rather, its presence is often in conjunction with other pulmonary problems.

Management
- The goal is to minimize inflation pressures and V_T.
- Use a mode that minimizes transpulmonary pressures (PIP, P_{alv}, PEEP) to minimize air leak through the fistula.
  - Minimize T_I, PIP (or V_T), P_{plat}, PEEP when possible
  - Minimize chest tube suction (may trigger ventilator)
- Ventilatory support should provide adequate inflation for the uninvolved areas of lung.
- Consider permissive hypercapnia to minimize inspiratory pressures and volumes.
- Management of oxygenation can be challenging since maneuvers that improve oxygenation (PEEP, T_I) also increase the leak
- Independent lung ventilation (see pg 9-43) and high-frequency jet ventilation (HFJV) have been used to address severe leak, although evidence (outcomes) doesn't support this. Surgical intervention may be indicated. ECMO may be indicated (VV or VA)

> The flow through a fistula is proportional to the magnitude and duration of the pressure gradient (e.g., P_{alv} 30 cmH_2O and chest tube suction - 20 cmH_2O = 50 cmH_2O pressure gradient).

Monitoring
- Careful monitoring of pressures and the volume of air leak (inspired V_T - expired V_T).

Weaning/Liberation
- Weaning strategy is based on the underlying disease process and closure of the air leak.

Diseases/Disorders

Burns (Thermal Injuries, Smoke Inhalation)

Injuries range from surface/skin burns (restrictive process) to inhalation injuries (thermal, smoke/toxic, and parenchymal). Carbon monoxide exposure is assumed if a fire.

Complications Associated with Burns and Smoke Inhalation:
- ARDS
- Airway obstruction
- CO poison
- Pneumonia
- Pulmonary edema
- Pulmonary embolism
- Sepsis
- Upper airway/ bronchial obstruction

Noninvasive Strategies
- NPPV is relatively contraindicated for burns.
- If CO poisoning is suspected or confirmed, CPAP (FIO_2 1.0) may be of benefit, assuming patient has stable level of consciousness.

Invasive Management
Indications for Mechanical Ventilation
- Surface Burns (especially if underlying ARDS), severe chest restriction, or respiratory depression (analgesia)
- Thermal injury if indications of thermal exposure (soot around nose/mouth) due to rapid onset of airway edema, spasm, and secretions.
- Exposure to toxins when respiratory depression (CO poisoning, cyanide, nitrogen oxides, etc.)
- Parenchymal injury when ARDS-like (smoke inhalation may paralyze mucociliary mechanism)

Suggested Ventilator Settings

V_T	6-8 mL/kg IBW
f	15-25 breaths/min (lower if auto-PEEP)
T_I	1.0 sec or less
PEEP	5 cmH$_2$O (start)
FIO$_2$	1.0 (especially in presence of carbon monoxide)

Management
- ARDS is a common development (see ARDS, page 9-2)
- Patients who are hypermetabolic may require high $\dot{V}_E$ to maintain CO$_2$ levels (normocarbia)
- If suspicion of CO exposure, use FIO$_2$ 1.0 until measured carboxyhemoglobin is below 10% (do not rely on PaO$_2$ or SpO$_2$)
- Repeated BALs may be indicated once sloughing occurs in thermal injuries
- Anticipate shifts in compliance/resistance (sloughing, scar tissue, etc.)

Monitoring
- Closely monitor for auto-PEEP if high $\dot{V}_E$ is used or patient exhibits bronchospasm and/or ↑ secretions.

Weaning/Liberation
- Reversal of the acute process usually leads to early and quick weaning, provided there are no secondary complications, such as ARDS, sepsis, or pulmonary infections.

Cardiac (Acute Events)
(MI, CHF)

This section covers two acute cardiac issues: myocardial infarction (MI) and acute cardiogenic pulmonary edema (ACPE). While presented together, the two have different clinical presentations and supportive needs.

- Severe heart failure can lead to hypoxia, increased work of breathing, and an increased work of the myocardium
- Causes include acute myocardial infarction (MI), fluid overload, hypertension, tachycardia (decreased fill time), and valvular diseases.

Cardiac Noninvasive Strategies

Myocardial Infarction
The use of NIV with an MI should only be considered with reservation. Any asynchrony or intolerance could add to the workload of the heart during a time when this may not be tolerated well.

Congestive Heart Failure
(acute cardiogenic pulmonary edema or ACPE)
- CPAP may help reduce preload, reduce left ventricular afterload, and prevent alveolar collapse at end-expiration
- NPPV should be considered if accompanying acute hypercapnia

Suggested Settings

CPAP	10-15 cmH$_2$O
FiO$_2$	1.0 (then wean down)

Cardiac Invasive Strategies

- In the presence of myocardial ischemia, choose modes that alleviate work of breathing (fuller support modes)
- Modes that risk increased WOB will increase oxygen demand, impacting on myocardia supply and demand.
- Spontaneous ventilation in patients with myocardial ischemia and high lung resistance and/or poor respiratory muscle function is likely detrimental.

Suggested Ventilator Settings

V_T	6-8 mL/kg IBW
f	$\geq$ 15 breaths/min
TI	$\leq$ 1 sec
Flow ($\dot{V}_I$)	> 60 L/min with decelerating pattern
PEEP	5-10 cmH$_2$O (monitor hemodynamics carefully)
FIO$_2$	1.0

Management
Initiate care with full support
Positive pressure ventilation (and increased pressures, such as through PEEP) decreases venous return. This can be therapeutic in some left ventricular dysfunction, but can be harmful if left ventricular function is normal.

Weaning/Liberation
- Weaning in cardiac patient is similar to exercise stress test. Careful monitoring must occur.
- Caution with PEEP titration (myocardial function is affected)
- Fluid balance and inotropes must be titrated concurrently to ensure maximum myocardial contractility.

Diseases/Disorders

Cardiac (Surgery, Post-Op)
(CABG)
Patients undergoing a coronary artery bypass graft surgery, and with some valve surgeries, qualify for a rapid wean post-surgery. The goal is early extubation.

A rapid weaning protocol (goal of extubation within several hours of arrival post-surgery) is utilized by many centers:

Suggested Settings

Mode	Varies, SIMV-VC is common
V_T	6-8 mL/kg IBW
f	10-12/min
PEEP	5-8 cmH$_2$O
FIO_2	0.50 (or per clinical need)
PSV	5-8 cmH$_2$O

Management
- Ensure ABG is within normal parameters (or at baseline)
- Sedation is weaned, then the ventilator (rate if using SIMV) is weaned to CPAP (with FIO_2 < 0.50)
- Ensure adequate respiratory parameters, hemodynamic stability, acid-base. If patient fails at any point, place back on full support, then retry after ~30 minutes.
- Underlying pulmonary conditions may complicate attempts to wean (COPD, asthma, obesity, etc.)

Chronic Obstructive Pulmonary Disease (COPD Exacerbation)

There are 3 symptoms that define a COPD exacerbation: increased dyspnea, increased sputum (or thicker viscosity), and increased sputum purulence. This is a change from baseline, which may result in the need to support oxygenation, ventilation, and work of breathing either noninvasively (preferred) or invasively (if necessary)

The need to provide support should be evaluated within the context of the patient's baseline.

Severity, by Clinical Signs*

Respiratory Failure	Absence of Failure	Non Life-Threatening	Life-Threatening
RR	20-30	> 30	> 30
PaO$_2$	improved with ≤ 35% O$_2$	improved with ≥ 35% O$_2$	requires ≥ 40% O$_2$
PaCO$_2$	No increase from baseline	Increased above baseline (or 50-60 torr)	Increased above baseline (or > 60 torr) (or pH ≤ 7.25)
Accessory Muscles	None	Yes, usually moderate	Yes, usually extensive
Mental Status	Baseline	Baseline	Acute change
Support	Baseline	NPPV	Invasive

* Adapted from COPD GOLD (2021)

Diseases/Disorders

COPD Noninvasive Strategies

There may be benefit to using NIV as a first-line intervention to reduce mortality and the need for intubation (when acute respiratory failure)*

Suggested Noninvasive Settings

Note: establish and document clinical goals, then titrate settings based on those.

NPPV	Generic settings to start: IPAP ~10 cmH$_2$O EPAP ~5 cmH$_2$O Titrate to clinical goals (CO$_2$, O$_2$, work of breathing) and tolerance
FiO$_2$	Goal is to keep FiO$_2$ < 0.50 when possible, but do not under treat clinical hypoxia

* Osadnik C, Tee V, Carson K, Wedzicha J, Smith B. Non-invasive ventilation for people with respiratory failure due to exacerbation of COPD. Cochrane reviews; 13 Jul 2017.

Once the patient can tolerate 4 hours of unassisted breathing, NPPV can be removed without further weaning (GOLD)

COPD Invasive Strategies
Indications for Intubation/Invasive Ventilation
See table on page 1-4, as well as:
- Diminished consciousness
- Inability to adequately control secretions
- Aspiration or vomiting
- Post-Respiratory or cardiac arrest
- Severe hemodynamic instability (or arrhythmias)

Suggested Settings

V_T	6-8 mL/kg IBW
f	8-16 breaths/min lower f may be needed to ensure full exhalation
T_I	0.6 - 1.2 sec lower TI may be needed to ensure full exhalation I:E ratio 1:4-1:6 is common
PEEP	5 cmH$_2$O PEEP to match 80% of measured auto-PEEP when triggering asynchrony noted
FiO$_2$	Maintain PaO$_2$ > 60 mmHg (or baseline clinical goal)
Flow ($\dot{V}_I$)	60 - 100 L/min with decelerating pattern

Monitoring
- Closely monitor for auto-PEEP (see pg 7-45)
- Clinical signs of cardiopulmonary distress (breath sounds, retractions, respiratory rate, etc.)
- Patient-ventilator asynchrony (trigger, etc.)

Diseases/Disorders

Management
- Decrease WOB to unload and rest ventilatory muscles (can take several days)
- Clinical goals should be to patient's baseline, not normalization of PCO_2, PaO_2
- Strategize to reduce Raw (bronchodilators, steroids, etc.)
- Assess and address anxiety, especially during weaning where baseline accessory muscles may have atrophied due to ventilator off-loading
- Secretions: monitor for hydration, mobilization, and clearance
- Nutrition: ensure balanced with set goal

Weaning/Liberation
- Wean when clinically improving
- Consider SBT with PSV over CPAP (or T-piece)
- Weaning can be challenging with severe COPD. Consider options to trial extubate to NPPV (even without perfect weaning parameters) or placement of a tracheostomy to facilitate weaning.

Drug Overdose and Poisoning

Clinical presentation of respiratory effect varies widely, ranging from minimal effect to complete respiratory and cardiac arrest.

ABC Considerations

Airway	If not patent, provide bag-mask ventilation. Consider naloxone if opioids are suspected. Intubate
Breathing	Severe metabolic acidosis is common (CO_2 may be extremely low. Be suspicious of normal CO_2 in these cases - risk of impending respiratory failure)
Circulation	Monitor for dysrhythmias (vary based on drug/poison). If hemodynamically unstable, intubation and ventilation likely necessary

- Attempts should be made to identify the cause or causes of overdose/toxicity (explore toxidromes: LOC, pupils, skin, motor tone, and vital signs)
- Ensure "scene" safety and anticipate sudden anxiety, restlessness, and combativeness
- Significant hyperthermia (> 40 C) and hypothermia (< 30 C) should be addressed (unless targeted temperature management)

Drug Overdose Noninvasive Strategies

Because of the risk of aspiration (including vomiting) and hemodynamic compromise, NIV strategies are relatively contraindicated and should only be considered in stable patients (with preference for high flow nasal interfaces over masks).

Invasive Strategies
Suggested Ventilator Settings

Settings are generally supportive (intubated for airway patency, ventilated for respiratory depression or tiring secondary to severe metabolic acidosis).

Mode	Full support mode (A/C, etc.) initially
V_T	6-8 mL/kg IBW
f	15-20 breaths/min Metabolic acidosis: increase $\dot{V}E$ to stabilize pH, but not cause auto-PEEP
TI	Normal, if higher f may need to decrease TI to allow for adequate TE
PEEP	5 cmH$_2$O
FIO$_2$	Varies by poison/drug. If in doubt, use higher FIO$_2$ until co-oximetry

Monitoring
- Aspiration pre-intubation is common with overdose
- Hemodynamic stability
- Level of consciousness,
- Patient-ventilator synchrony may be significant challenge

Weaning/Liberation
- Allow time for drugs to be metabolized and eliminated. Be aware of factors that slow this (renal and hepatic function, obesity, metabolic rates, etc.)
- The patient may have periods of alertness followed by decreased LOC. Ensure careful backup settings in spontaneous modes.
- Assess for underlying neurologic deficits, aspiration injury, etc.
- Anticipate challenges in weaning/discontinuation in patients with underlying addictions (and now withdrawal)

Neuromuscular Disorders

Clinical presentation of respiratory effect varies widely, ranging from minimal effect to complete respiratory and cardiac arrest.

Types

While myasthenia gravis and Guillain Barré syndrome are more common critical care disorders, there are various others:

Rapid Onset (days to weeks)	Gradual Onset (months to years)
Botulism	ALS
Cervical spinal cord injury	Muscular dystrophy
Guillain Barré Syndrome	Post polio syndrome
Myasthenia gravis	Progressive thoracic deformities
Tetanus	

Monitoring

- Closely monitor pulmonary mechanics (V_T, FVC, NIF). When deterioration beyond acceptable levels, consider options. V_T or FVC deficiency may benefit from NIV, but a decreased NIF may indicate need for airway patency (intubation)
- Dyspnea and abnormal sputum are typical presentations with chronic neuromuscular disease. However, distress may appear less than the actual clinical state (unable to cough effectively, unable to increase minute ventilation independently). Check acid-base, careful physical assessment.

Neuromuscular Noninvasive Strategies

- Early initiation of NIV in critical care may help prevent intubation (GBS is an exception). Assess airway patency (including secretion management) carefully.
- Clinical goals may include improvement of FRC, support of tidal volume when weakness.
- Titrate V_T to goal (~8 mL/kg IBW)

Diseases/Disorders

Neuromuscular Invasive Ventilator Settings

Some clinicians suggest initiating invasive support using the 20/30/40 rule: VC < 20 mL/kg, NIF > -30 cmH$_2$O, MEP < 40 cmH$_2$O

Suggested Ventilator Settings

Mode	The choice between full and partial support varies by disorder, but if an acute process with a chronic disorder, consider full support
V$_T$	Acute: consider lung protective (6-8 mL/kg IBW) Chronic: VT at a higher range (8+ mL)
f	Maintain adequate minute ventilation
T$_I$	≤ 1 sec
Flow ($\dot{V}_I$)	≤ 60 L/min (normal lung volumes) ≥ 60 L/min (reduced lung volumes)
PEEP	5 cmH$_2$O (maintain FRC)
FIO$_2$	Should be minimal once lungs are recruited

Management

- The main needs of these patients are adequate lung inflation and appropriate airway clearance. Provide support based on the patient's inherent ventilatory muscle strengths.
- Psychologically some of these patients desire or demand large V$_T$, high flow, fast rates, and long T$_I$ (more than needed). Adjust to satisfy patient's inspiratory needs.

Weaning/Liberation

- Primary acute process should be reversed, unless new chronic process
- Goal: return to baseline settings. Additional ICU weakness of muscles may complicate weaning

Postoperative Management

Patients needing post-op management due to anesthesia, instability that requires continued mechanical ventilation

Postoperative Noninvasive Strategies

Once extubated, initiating noninvasive support is indicated in patients who use noninvasive therapy at home (obstructive sleep apnea)

Postoperative Invasive Strategies
Suggested Ventilator Settings

V_T	6-8 mL/kg IBW
f	12-20 breaths/min
T_I	Normal Range
PEEP	5 cmH$_2$O
FIO$_2$	Should be minimal if no underlying issues

Management
- Avoid healthcare complications: infection, decreased cardiac output, hyperventilation, inspissated secretions, and exposure to unnecessary supplemental oxygen
- Assess within the context of any comorbidities which might complicate clearance of anesthesia (obesity, renal failure, hepatic dysfunction) and weaning (COPD, asthma, etc.)

Restrictive Disorders

This group of disorders includes thoracic cage abnormalities like kyphoscoliosis; a component of progressive neuromuscular disorders like ALS; and may also include obesity-related syndromes. Severity varies widely.

Restrictive Disorders Noninvasive Strategies

- NPPV may successfully treat hypoventilation aspects, preventing or alleviating respiratory fatigue
- Some patients at baseline require overnight support, but may have an increased need during an acute process

Restrictive Disorders Invasive Strategies
Suggested Ventilator Settings

V_T	6-8 mL/kg IBW
f	12-30 breaths/min (increased to maintain ↑ $\dot{V}_E$)
T_I	≤ 1.0 sec
Flow ($\dot{V}_I$)	≥ 60 L/min with decelerating waveform
PEEP	5 cmH$_2$O (maintain FRC) Higher PEEP levels may be considered to offset chest wall restrictions, such as with obesity
FIO$_2$	As needed to meet oxygenation goals

Diseases/Disorders

Trauma (Chest)

Two generalized categories are blunt chest trauma and penetrating traumas. The possible cause of trauma is an endless list, ranging from accidental (vehicle crash, etc.) to violent (stabbing, gunshot) to industrial (crush injury, etc.)

Basic Types and Strategies

Blunt Chest Traumas	
Pulmonary Contusion	Irregular opacification on CXR Creates areas of V/Q mismatch (oxygenation may be difficult, position with good lung down) Resolve in ~1 week Goal is to control pain, ensure adequate airway clearance Watch for pneumonia, ARDS, common complications
Pneumothorax	Active air leak: Depending on severity, V_{TE} will decrease (air exits through the pneumothorax instead of back through ventilator)
Rib Fractures	Pain control If severe, analgesia may reduce respiratory drive (intubate) Flail segment (2 or more adjacent rib fractures with 2 or more breaks per rib): NPPV may be appropriate to stabilize. If decompensation, may need to be intubated
Penetrating Traumas	
Low-velocity (stabbings) **Medium-velocity** (handgun) **High-velocity** (rifles, military)	Risk of tension pneumothorax (acute hypotension, unilateral chest rise) Risk of cardiac injury Surgical intervention may be required - post-op management

Chest Trauma Noninvasive Strategies

- NIV may be helpful for patients who are shallow-breathing due to underlying pain (CPAP) or have mild respiratory distress (NPPV), assuming the airway is patent and the respiratory drive (especially with analgesia) is intact. Avoid with pneumothorax until stabilized.
- May help stabilize chest, preventing intubation
- Consider a low threshold for intubation, particularly if hemodynamic involvement or deteriorating P/F ratio

Noninvasive Suggested Settings

Mode	CPAP (5-10 cmH$_2$O) for stabilization NPPV (EPAP 5-10 with IPAP set for desired V$_T$) for stabilization + respiratory distress
FIO$_2$	If low lung volumes (atelectasis due to hypoventilation), low FIO2 needed after initial recruitment

Chest Trauma Invasive Strategies

Suggested Ventilator Settings

Mode	Complete protective/supportive approach
V$_T$	6-8 mL/kg IBW (normal compliance) 4-8 mL/kg IBW (pulmonary contusions)
f	15-25 breaths/min
TI	≤ 1.0 sec
PEEP	5 cmH$_2$O Use caution with PEEP in presence of air leaks
FIO$_2$	Start at 1.0, then wean for clinical goal (PaO$_2$ ~60-80 torr)

Management
- Pain management can be challenging (uncontrolled pain can lead to increased O_2 consumption, work of breathing, atelectasis from guarded breathing; oversedation can lead to respiratory depression)
- Lung protective strategies are indicated to prevent further injury to the lungs
- If risk of pneumothorax: use lowest mean airway pressure (including PEEP) possible to maintain clinical stability

Monitoring
- Air leak
- Atelectasis
- Pulmonary embolism
- Hemodynamic instability
- Pneumonia (most common complication)

Weaning/Liberation
- Discontinuation often occurs early and rapidly unless ARDS develops or severe chest wall or diaphragm injury is present.

Trauma (Head)

This topic covers unexpected bleeds, traumatic injuries, tumors, etc. Critical care involves careful monitoring of ICP and CPP, which are sensitive to ventilator settings and respiratory management (suctioning, intubation, etc.)

Types
- Intracerebral Hemorrhage:
  - Subarachnoid Hemorrhage (SAH)
  - Subdural Hematoma (SDH)
  - Intraventricular Hemorrhage (IVH)
- Diffuse Axonal Injury (DAI)
- Cerebral Contusion
- Concussion

Patient Problems: Cerebral edema and/or ↑ ICP

CPP = MAP - ICP	CPP > 120 mmHg = encephalopathy, cerebral edema
	Normal CPP = 50-70 mmHg
	CPP < 50 = poor perfusion

CPP = Cerebral Perfusion Pressure (mmHg)
MAP = Mean Arterial Pressure (mmHg) ... Normal = 70-80 mmHg
ICP = Intracranial Pressure (mmHg) ... Normal = < 15 mmHg

Common Causes

- Stroke (CVA)
- Hepatic failure
- Post-resuscitation hypoxia
- Surgery (post craniotomy)
- Trauma

Invasive Ventilator Management
Indications for Invasive Ventilation
- Central respiratory depression from injury or drugs used to treat acute head injury (barbiturate coma, sedation, paralysis)
- Glasgow Coma Score (GCS)
- Abnormal (or worsened) sputum production (amount, color, consistency) 8
- Impending or actual cardiac arrest
- Neurogenic pulmonary edema

Suggested Ventilator Settings

Mode	Mode/Settings that minimize the risk of asynchrony or patient effort (may require sedation)
V_T	8 mL/kg IBW*
f	10-15 breaths/min*
T_I	≤ 1.0 sec
Flow ($\dot{V}_I$)	High (keep T_I short)
PEEP	≤ 5 cmH$_2$O *PEEP increases the intrathoracic pressure, preventing some venous return from the head (leading to an increased ICP). Careful application of PEEP and subsequent monitoring is critical.*
F_IO_2	Use 1.0 initially *Hypoxemia may contribute further to injury (ensure PaO$_2$ > 60 torr, some use higher target of 80-100)*

* Maintain PaCO$_2$ between 32-45 mmHg (improves outcomes). This can be done through a combination of increasing the set rate and using a V_T that is on the high end of normal (~8 mL/kg iBW)

Ventilator Management
- Positive pressure ventilation and PEEP can ↑ ICP because Palv is easily transmitted to vascular space in patients with normal lungs.
- Monitor for and address auto-PEEP
- Suctioning may induce a Valsalva response. Only suction when clear indications (secretions are affecting clinical status)
- Patient sedation is critical: avoid metabolic demand, ventilator asynchrony, and tachycardia (propofol is recommended)

Brain Trauma Foundation Guidelines (4th ed)

Respiratory Recommendations
- Prophylactic prolonged hyperventilation (PaCO$_2$ ≤ 25) is not recommended
- Early tracheostomy is recommended to reduce ventilator days (weigh risks vs. benefits), although there's no evidence that it reduces mortality or rate of pneumonia
- Avoid use of povidone-iodine oral care (to reduce VAP) as it may increase risk of ARDS
- Avoid use of aggressive fluids/pressors to maintain CPP > 70 mmHg due to risk of respiratory failure

Other respiratory recommendations that have been formally de-emphasized due to lack of evidence, but are still included:

- Avoid hyperventilation in the first 24 hours after injury
- Hyperventilation is recommended as a temporizing measure for lowering increased ICP
- If hyperventilation is used, monitor O$_2$ delivery with jugular venous O$_2$ Sat (SJO$_2$) or brain tissue O$_2$ tension (PbrO$_2$)

In addition, recommendations not directly related to ventilator management, but relevant to care include:

- BP: maintain systolic 100+ mmHg 50-69 years-old or 110+ for all others.
- ICP (treat if above 22 mmHg) and CPP (target 60-70 mmHg as minimum optimal) monitoring is an important component of guiding the management of a TBI
- AVDO$_2$ (maintain < 50%) monitoring should be considered
- Targeted temperature management (prophylactic hypothermia) is not recommended for short-term care
- Avoid high-dose propofol for management (increases morbidity). Barbiturates may be necessary to control elevated ICPs that are refractory to treatment.
- The use of steroids is contraindicated (should be avoided in their use to reduce ICP)

*These recommendations are summarized from the Guidelines for the Management of Severe Traumatic Brain Injury, 4th Edition, 2016. BrainTrauma.org. They were a joint project of the Brain Trauma Foundation, AANS, CNS, and the AANS/CNS Joint Section on Neurotrauma and Critical Care

Diseases/Disorders

ICP Evaluation and Management

Monitor for symptoms of elevated ICP:
- Cushing triad: bradycardia, respiratory depression, hypertension (may all indicate brain stem compression, controversial)
- Headache
- Vomiting
- Change in level of consciousness
- Periorbital bruising

Management
- Minimize any further elevations in ICP:
  - Patient positioning during intubation (avoid excessive flexion)
  - Careful choice of RSI
  - Consider use of lidocaine in pretreatment
- **Hyperventilation** ($PaCO_2$ 26-30 mmHg) may be cautiously considered with cerebral edema, intracranial hemorrhage, and some tumors as an urgent intervention for increased ICP.
  - Hyperventilation reduces ICP through vasoconstriction (1 mmHg decrease in $PaCO_2$ reduces cerebral blood flow by 3%)
  - Avoid use of hyperventilation with TBI or CVA (may worsen the underlying neurological injury by decreasing cerebral perfusion)
- Avoid hypotension (especially with hypoxemia) as reactive vasodilation and elevations in ICP can occur
- Avoid severe fluid restrictions

Weaning/Liberation
- Extubating patients with underlying brain trauma should be considered a higher-risk decision. While not to be delayed, plans for reintubation should be in place due to the higher risk of extubation failure.
- Careful consideration for weaning in patients with diminished mental status (ensure airway protective reflexes, adequate ventilatory drive, etc.). GCS > 10 is recommended. Ability to track visually is recommended.
- Consider fluid balance (negative is preferred)

Diseases/Disorders

Unilateral Disorders

This section covers a generic category of disorders that affect one lung, or sometimes one region of one lung (pneumonia, severe contusion, lung abscess, lung transplantation, etc.).

It is important to consider the underlying mechanics of a unilateral process. Air will preferentially follow the path of least resistance, the more compliant lung. This may over-ventilate (pneumonia, etc.) the healthy lung.

Unilateral Disorders Invasive Strategies
Suggested Ventilator Settings

V_T	6-8 mL/kg IBW
f	12-20 breaths/min (increased to maintain $\uparrow \dot{V}_E$)
T_I	≤ 1.0 sec
Flow ($\dot{V}_I$)	≥ 60 L/min with decelerating waveform
PEEP	5+ cmH$_2$O May be used therapeutically to recruit lung
FIO$_2$	As needed to meet oxygenation goals

Management
- Treat the underlying infection when possible
- Consider patient positioning to optimize V/Q
  - Bad Lung Up, Good Lung Down
  - If infectious process, bleeding: Good Lung Up, Bad Lung Down (avoid draining infectious secretions into good lung)
- Severe unilateral process: consider independent lung ventilation (ventilate the "good" lung and the "bad" lung separately) - see next page - or potentially ECMO

Independent Lung Ventilation (ILV)

Indications
Consider when there are difficulties with conventional ventilation
- Aspiration
- Hemoptysis (massive)
- Lung abscess
- Lung contusions
- Lung transplantation (single)
- Pneumonia (severe)
- Pulmonary edema/hemorrhage (unilateral)

Basic Procedure
- Intubate with a dual lumen endotracheal tube:
  - Distal lumen sits in bronchus (usually left)
    cuff on lumen isolates lung where it sits
  - Proximal lumen sits in trachea
    cuff on lumen seals lower airway from upper airway
- Placement should be verified by bronchoscopy
- Two ventilators are generally utilized in one of two ways:
  - Synchronous: lungs are ventilated in some coordination with each other. This requires an electronic cable to join two ventilators together (available with some ventilators)
  - Dyssynchronous: lungs are ventilated independently

Suggested Settings*

Parameter	Healthy Lung	Unhealthy Lung
Mode	A/C	CPAP or A/C
V_T total: 6 mL/kg IBW	< 5 mL/kg IBW	minimal (Pplat < 30)
PEEP	~5 cmH$_2$O	optimal PEEP (usually more than healthy lung)
FiO$_2$	Per PaO$_2$ goal	Low (~ 30%)

Once stabilization/improvement, wean settings of unhealthy lung towards settings of healthy lung. Once settings match, consider transition back to single lumen ET tube

*Berg S. Independent lung ventilation: implementation strategies and review of literature. World J Crit Care Med. 2019:Jul 31:8(4)49-58

Diseases/Disorders

Viral Pulmonary Disorders (COVID, etc.)

While COVID became a focal point for critical care strategies, the underlying strategy is similar for most viral disorders: slow down the virus replication if possible (antivirals), then support oxygenation and ventilation until symptoms improve.

- While signs and symptoms vary by patient (and especially with comorbid conditions), many patients with viral pulmonary disorders present with hypoxemic respiratory failure (without significant hypercapnia)

Suggested Noninvasive Settings

Mode	<ul><li>HFOT/CPAP may help prevent intubation in some patients with oxygenation issues</li><li>HFNC, in particular, may be more tolerated with some patients</li><li>NPPV is indicated in patients with increased work of breathing, worsening respiratory acidosis</li></ul>
HFNC	Set flow rate (25-35 L/min to start), can titrate up to 60 L/min per tolerance/clinical effect
CPAP NPPV	Consider use of higher CPAP (or EPAP, ensuring adequate ΔP IPAP-EPAP) levels when hypoxemic respiratory failure. This is preferred (if tolerated) over higher FIO$_2$ levels.
FIO$_2$	Maintain minimum goals with preference to optimizing flow rates or CPAP/EPAP first.

- Consider lower goals for oxygenation (SpO$_2$ > 93% during resuscitation; > 89% during maintenance)
- Monitor respiratory status closely. If no improvement or worsening (mental status, refractory hypoxemia, increased work of breathing) consider intubation
- Some patients benefit from alternating between HFNC when awake, then transitioning to NPPV by mask when asleep

Invasive Strategies
Suggested Ventilator Settings

Mode	Full support initially. As with most disorders, optimizing settings is more important than which modes is selected.
V_T	6-8 mL/kg IBW Lung protective if evidence of ARDS
f	10-15 breaths/min May need to increase if pH worsens
TI	Ensure adequate exhalation time, especially at higher rate
PEEP	Higher PEEPs may be trialed with hypoxemic respiratory failure Optimize PEEP (see page 7-26)
FiO_2	Use 1.0 initially

Management
- **With all infectious processes, care should be provided in a way that minimizes transmission to others, including the clinician** (intubation, suctioning, ventilator circuit care, bronchoscopy, extubation, etc.)
- It is reasonable to consider patient positioning (good lung down if unilateral process, prone if bilateral) early when hypoxemic (and cause of hypoxemia is likely the viral infection)
- Assess for patient-ventilator synchrony often. Asynchrony will increase oxygen consumption, which can be detrimental with severe hypoxemic respiratory failure (NMBAs may be indicated).
- During the acute phase of illness, oxygenation (and sometimes ventilation) may be challenging (life-threatening, in some cases). Consider minimum acceptable clinical goals (SpO_2 > 93% during resuscitation; > 89% during maintenance), pH > 7.25, for example, versus normalization.

Diseases/Disorders

- Consider alternative strategies early (proning, including on noninvasive), inhaled prostaglandins, etc.
- Note comorbid conditions that could complicate care (ensuring appropriate drug therapy for COPD, for example)

Weaning/Discontinuation

- Consider SBT by a closed system (avoid T-piece trials due to infection transmission risks) once symptoms improve
- Use additional precaution with extubation of known difficult airways (the risk of reintubation increases transmission risks)
- Postextubation clinical targets are similar to preintubation clinical targets. Consider use of HFOT, NIV, etc.

10 Ventilator Effects

Pulmonary
- Airway Obstruction 10-2
- Atelectasis/Derecruitment 10-3
- Auto-PEEP (Air Trapping) 10-4
- Hyperoxic Lung Injury (Toxicity) 10-8
- Respiratory Drive (Decreased) 10-9
- Ventilation/Perfusion Imbalance 10-10
- Work of Breathing 10-11
- Lung Injury 10-12
- Hypoventilation 10-14
- Hyperventilation 10-15

Extrapulmonary
- Cardiac 10-16
- Neurological 10-16
- Nutritional 10-17
- Hepatic 10-17
- Gastrointestinal 10-17
- Renal 10-17

Ventilator-Associated Infections
- Ventilator-Associated Events 10-19
- VAE/VAP Bundle 10-20

Pulmonary Effects

Airway Obstruction

Causes	Patient	• Bronchoconstriction • Inadequate airway clearance (suctioning, therapies)
	Circuit	• ET (or trach) tube displaced, kinked, or cuff herniated • Water/secretions in circuit
Signs & Symptoms	Patient	• Adventitious breath sounds • ↓ PaO_2 • ↑ WOB
	Vent	• ↑ PIP (volume modes) • ↓ volumes (pressure modes) (pressure limited volumes) • Patient-ventilator asynchrony
Strategies	• Systematically identify the cause of the obstruction, then address it	

Atelectasis/Derecruitment

Causes	Patient	<ul><li>Underlying disease/disorder (consolidation, etc.)</li><li>Inadequate airway clearance (mucous plugs, etc.)</li><li>Excessive supplemental oxygen (nitrogen washout)</li></ul>
	Vent	<ul><li>Low V_T</li><li>Sub-optimal PEEP</li><li>High FiO_2 (absorption atelectasis)</li></ul>
Signs & Symptoms	Patient	<ul><li>Diminished breath sounds</li><li>Fine crackles</li><li>$\downarrow SpO_2$ and PaO_2</li><li>Chest imaging consistent with atelectasis/low lung volumes</li></ul>
	Vent	<ul><li>↑ PIP (volume modes)</li><li>↓ V_T (pressure modes)</li></ul>
Strategies		<ul><li>Systematically identify the cause, correct if able (bronchoscopy for significant secretions, etc.)</li><li>Use recruitment strategies to improve (PEEP optimization, recruitment maneuver, patient positioning, etc.)</li></ul>

Effects

Auto-PEEP (Air Trapping)

unintentional PEEP during mechanical ventilation when inspiration begins before exhalation is complete, resulting in air trapped in the lungs.

Causes	Patient	↑ **Expiratory Raw or airway collapse on exhalation:** • Ball-valve obstruction • Bronchospasm • COPD (collapse) • Mucosal edema • Secretions **Active exhalation (no air-trapping)** • Increased $\dot{V}E$ (pain, fever, ARDS)
	Vent	**Inadequate Expiratory Time:** • Long TI • Slow $\dot{V}I$ • High f • High/Inverse I:E ratio **Mechanical expiratory Raw:** • ET tube • Exhalation valve, PEEP valve
Signs & Symptoms	Patient	• ↑A-P Diameter (barrel chest) • ↑ Radiolucency on CXR • ↑ Resonance on percussion • ↑ WOB
	Vent	• Graphics (see below) • ↑ PIP in volume modes • ↑ P$_{Plat}$ • ↓ Synchrony

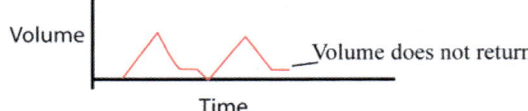

Effects

Clinical Effects	<ul><li>Alveolar overdistension</li><li>Flattened hemidiaphragms</li><li>Hemodynamic compromise</li><li>Patient-Ventilator asynchrony</li><li>↓ Compliance</li><li>↓ Efficiency of pulmonary muscles</li><li>↑ Effort to trigger ventilator</li><li>↑ Risk of volutrauma</li></ul>	
Identifying (Known)	1. *Flow / time curve*: **Expiratory flow fails to return to zero before next inspiration begins (see below)** 2. *Respirometer*: Connect a respirometer to patient's ET tube. The needle is moving when next inspiration begins.	
Identifying (Suspected)	Patient	<ul><li>Accessory muscle use/paradoxical breathing</li><li>↓ BS, ↓ chest wall movement</li><li>Dyspnea/discomfort</li><li>CXR: ↑ radiolucency, flattened hemidiaphragms</li><li>Inspiratory efforts do not trigger ventilator</li><li>JVD during exhalation (collapse during inspiration)</li><li>Patient exhaling when next breath starts</li><li>Prolonged time constant</li><li>Patient's RR > ventilator response rate (assumes sensitivity is set properly)</li></ul>
	Ventilator	<ul><li>↑ PIP and P_{plat}</li><li>Transient ↓ in exhaled V_T's</li><li>High ventilator rates (AC)</li></ul>

Effects

Measuring Auto-PEEP

End-Expiratory Pause	• The exhalation valve is occluded for 1 – 2 sec. (some up to 4 sec) just prior to next inspiration; inspiration is delayed. • As Palv equilibrates with the proximal Paw, the level of auto-PEEP is reflected on the pressure gauge during the pause (accuracy is questionable). • Auto-PEEP = total PEEP – set PEEP • $PEEP_I = PEEP_{tot} - PEEP_E$
T-Piece Adapter (Braschi Valve)	• A T-piece adaptor with a one-way valve and cap. • The cap is removed during exhalation. • While the next mechanical breath is diverted out the uncapped hole, the pressure equilibrates between the patient's lungs and circuit. • Auto-PEEP pressure is read on a manometer proximal to the patient.
Pplat Estimate	• Measure P_{plat} during volume ventilation (P_{plat} #1) • Place on CPAP for 30 sec • Return to Volume Mode and measure P_{plat} on 1st or 2nd breath (P_{plat} # 2) • (P_{plat} 1) – (P_{plat} 2) = rough estimate of auto-PEEP

Clinical Note: Measuring auto-PEEP by end-expiratory pressure requires a quiet patient with no spontaneous breathing and a circuit with no leaks.
Many ventilators have a function that directly measure auto-PEEP.

Effects

Considerations to Reduce Auto-PEEP

1. Increase Expiratory Time (TE) by:
- Decreasing Rate (↑ TE)
- Decreasing VT (↓ TI)
- Decreasing Inspiratory Time
- Increasing Flow (↓ TI)

2. Airflow Obstruction
- Administer SABAs
- Airway clearance (lavage? therapeutic bronchoscopy?)
- Steroid administration
- Consider changing to larger ET Tube

3. Decrease Minute Ventilation
- Manage pain
- Treat fever
- Use of sedation if clinically indicated

4. Allow as much spontaneous breathing as possible:
- Pressure support ventilation (with adequate support)
- CPAP (less common, PSV is preferred)
- SIMV (may increase asynchrony so assess closely)

5. Apply PEEP/CPAP (see page 7-29)
Carefully ↑ applied PEEP in increments of 1 cmH₂O until the patient's rate and the ventilator rate are equal. (Applied PEEP > auto-PEEP may lead to further hyperinflation and complications).

6. Lower resistance exhalation valve (if available)

Clinical Note: Permissive hypercapnia is sometimes recommended when auto-PEEP cannot be reduced due to high $\dot{V}_E$ demand and/or severe airway obstruction.

Hyperoxic Lung Injury (Oxygen Toxicity)

Causes	Higher amounts of supplemental oxygen over time. The exact amounts are unclear, but giving over 50% for > 48-hours increases risk. This excess oxygen has known effects: vasoconstriction, cytokine release, etc. Highest levels of O_2 (close to 100%) may cause absorption atelectasis (as nitrogen normally keeps alveoli open, with O_2 being a poor replacement as it quickly diffuses over the A/C membrane)
Signs & Symptoms	Symptoms similar to bronchitis: • ↓ PaO_2 with ↑ $P(A-a)O_2$ • ↓ Compliance • ↑ V/Q mismatch
Strategies	• Wean O_2 aggressively until < 50% when clinical goals are being met • Consider lower oxygenation targets when clinically appropriate (such as with ARDS)

Respiratory Drive Decreased

Causes	<ul><li>Overventilation (rate on vent exceeds patient's physiological need)</li><li>Sedation (or sedation with paralytics)</li><li>Drug overdose</li><li>Underlying neurological condition</li></ul>
Signs & Symptoms	<ul><li>Apnea* in spontaneous modes (or decrease in spontaneous triggering)</li><li>Insufficiency will lead to ↑ $PaCO_2$, ↓ PaO_2</li><li>Hypocapnia (rate set too high on ventilator, patient is "riding" the vent rate)</li></ul>
Strategies	<ul><li>This may be the therapeutic goal to allow patient to minimize O_2 consumption, etc.</li><li>Systematically assess cause of decrease (sedation bolus, vent settings, etc.), then decide how to proceed</li></ul>

* This may particularly be noted when switching suddenly to a spontaneous mode (PSV) from A/C with a high ventilator rate. The patient has no drive to breathe until their CO_2 has had a chance to rise adequately. This, at times, is mistaken for weaning failure.

Ventilation/Perfusion (V/Q) Imbalances

Causes	<ul><li>The relationship of ventilation (flow of air) and perfusion (flow of blood) affects gas exchange efficiency</li><li>V/Q imbalances are complex and dependent on a patient's pathophysiology and the level/mode of ventilation. See table on bottom of page for examples</li></ul>
Signs & Symptoms	<ul><li>Refractory hypoxemia</li><li>Hypercapnia</li><li>Confusion/somnolence</li></ul>

Strategies	1. **Strategically position the patient**
	  Place Bad Lung Up, Good Lung Down
	  (BLU GLD, or Blue Gold)
	  (unless infectious secretions in bad lung, then reverse this)
	  Trial prone position to optimize $\dot{V}/Q$
	2. **Optimize alveolar recruitment**
	  (the ventilation side of $\dot{V}/Q$)
	  Lung expansion, CPAP, PEEP, etc.
	3. **Ensure adequate perfusion**
	  Pulmonary vasodilators, minimize O_2 (which causes vasoconstriction), etc.

Ventilation exceeds perfusion	Perfusion exceeds ventilation
Ventilation with reduced or no perfusion = dead space	**Perfusion with reduced or no ventilation = shunt**
V/Q > 0.8	V/Q < 0.8
<ul><li>Heart failure</li><li>Pulmonary embolus</li><li>Emphysema</li><li>Pulmonary capillary damage</li></ul>	<ul><li>Airway obstruction</li><li>ARDS</li><li>Atelectasis</li><li>Aspiration</li><li>Asthma (severe)</li><li>Pneumonia</li><li>Pulmonary edema</li></ul>

Work of Breathing (WOB)

Causes	Patient	<ul><li>↓ C (various)</li><li>High inspiratory flow demand (various)</li><li>↑ Raw (various)</li></ul>
	Circuit	<ul><li>Inadequate $\dot{V}_I$</li><li>Insensitive trigger</li><li>Inadequate demand valve (SIMV)</li><li>High resistance circuits, ET tubes, humidifiers, PEEP, and/or exhalation valves.</li></ul>
Signs & Symptoms	Patient	<ul><li>Accessory muscle use</li><li>↑ Spontaneous rate</li><li>Restlessness/anxiety</li><li>Nasal flaring</li><li>Diaphoresis</li><li>Retractions</li></ul>
	Machine	<ul><li>Asynchrony</li><li>↑ PIP</li></ul>
Strategies	\multicolumn{2}{l	}{<ul><li>Address any underlying causes<ul><li>Pain management</li><li>Inadequate sedation</li><li>Anxiety/delirium</li><li>Fever</li><li>Hypoxemia</li></ul></li><li>Ensure patient-ventilator synchrony (settings, mode) (see pg 7-45 to 7-50)</li><li>Decrease airway resistance (see pg 4-14)</li><li>Increase lung compliance (see pg 4-13)</li></ul>}

Lung Injury

Ventilator-Induced Lung Injury	VILI	acute lung injury caused by (or worsened by) the ventilator
Ventilator-Associated Lung Injury	VALI	injury not proven to be caused by the ventilator (could also be due to underlying condition of the lungs)
Self-Induced Lung Injury	SILI	injury caused at least in part by spontaneous tidal volumes
Signs & Symptoms	\multicolumn{2}{l}{Worsening hypoxemia Worsening compliance Increased O_2 needs Respiratory distress CXR: new opacities}

Mechanisms of Injury
See damage cascade, next page, for details

Volutrauma (overdistension):
High volumes cause overdistension of alveoli in higher compliance areas (generally a VT above ~6 mL/kg IBW increases risk, but it is important to remember that a disproportionate volume is delivered to the higher compliance areas ... the open alveoli). Use of lung protective strategies will decrease risk.

Atelectrauma:
Damage caused by the repeated expansion (inspiration) and collapse (expiration) of alveoli, creating shear forces that cause injury to alveoli and airways. Surfactant deficiency (such as with ARDS) may further complicate this. PEEP may help prevent this when optimized.

Biotrauma (inflammation):
Inflammatory mediators are released from injured lungs (this can be caused by volutrauma and atelectrauma). Corticosteroids may be of benefit to some patients.

Effects

Damage begins a cascade of:

> Trauma → Air Leak → ↑Vascular Permeability → Fluid/Protein shifts across A-C Membrane → High Permeability Pulmonary Edema → Surfactant Disturbance → Alveolar Instability → ↓ C → V/Q Mismatch → Shunting → ↓ Gas Exchange → Activated immunological response → Release of Inflammatory Mediators (Cytokines) → Neutrophil Aggregation → Fibrin Deposits → Fibrotic Changes → Widened Air/Blood Interface → ↓ FRC → Systemic Inflammatory Response (SIRS) → ↑ Morbidity and Mortality

Lung Protective Strategies

Reduce Positive Pressure Ventilation	• Minimize potentially damaging pressures
	  • Minimize PPlat (< 30 cmH$_2$O)
	  • Low VT (6-8 mL/kg IBW) (prevent overdistension)
	• Permissive hypoxemia (minimize mechanical effects of vent)
	• Permissive hypercapnia (minimize mechanical effects of vent)
	• Rapid weaning (minimize time on vent)

Open Lung Approach	• Adequate PEEP (minimize shearing, prevent derecruitment, maximize ventilation) • Lung recruitment (overcome the closing pressure and minimize threshold opening pressure of collapsed alveoli): • Sustained inflation
Alternative Strategies	• Use of NMBAs (for severe breath-stacking, for example) • Prone positioning (when V/Q mismatch) • ECMO (decreases mechanical stresses of being on a ventilator) • High-frequency ventilation (HFOV)

Effects

Hypoventilaton

Causes	Patient	↑ $\dot{V}_E$ demand
	Vent	Settings below minute ventilation needed
Signs & Symptoms	Patient	↑ $PaCO_2$ with ↓ pH ↑ WOB May lead to: • Decreased PaO_2 (or increasing O_2 need) • Hyperkalemia • Increased ICP in patients with brain dysfunction • Right-shift of oxygen-hemoglobin dissociation curve

> Hypercapnia with moderate acidosis is not as harmful as high level ventilation to maintain normal CO_2.
> Rapid ↑ $PaCO_2$ and ↓ pH can lead to coma.

Effects

Hyperventilation

Causes	Patient	↓ $\dot{V}_E$ demand Hypoxia
	Machine	↑ $\dot{V}_E$ delivered
Signs & Symptoms	Patient	↓ $PaCO_2$ with ↑ pH May lead to: • Lung injury • ↓ Cardiac output • Hypokalemia • Left-shift of oxygen-hemoglobin dissociation curve

Prolonged, severe hypocapnia can lead to tetany and ↓ cerebral perfusion. Normal CO_2 levels in chronic CO_2 retainers may indicate relative hyperventilation.

Effects

Extrapulmonary Effects

Cardiac *effects more pronounced with higher lung compliance* *ensure optimized settings* *use of drugs (pressors, etc.) may be indicated*	
↓ CO (hypotension)	Caused in part by decreased venous return and diminished ventricular output PEEP (and auto-PEEP) contribute to this (consider PEEP levels) This can be used therapeutically in some patients with left ventricular failure
↑ PVR	Complex relationship (alveolar pressures constrict pulmonary vasculature, etc.), most with right ventricular failure Both derecruitment and hyperexpansion can increase PVR (optimize settings, especially PEEP)
False hemodynamic values	Values taken at end-expiration are most likely to be effected (PEEP influence) PCWP may be falsely elevated Estimate: Subtract 1/2 of PEEP level (normal C) or 1/4 of PEEP level (low C) from PCWP
Neurological *effects more pronounced if ICP elevated due to injury/surgery*	
↑ ICP ↓ CPP	Intrathoracic pressures can decrease venous return from the head Increased risk of ischemia
Neuro-inflammation	Evidence suggests alveolar stretching and hyperoxic lung injury triggers an inflammatory response, resulting in damage of the brain Lung protective strategies may decrease risk

Nutritional	
ensure careful feeding targets	
Overfeeding (above target)	Can result in excess CO_2 production, increased WOB May complicate weaning as body has to eliminate excess CO_2 being produced Consider calorimetry with careful goal setting
Underfeeding (below target)	May lead to additional muscle weakness and atrophy Increased risk of complications (PE, pneumonia, etc.)
Hepatic	
monitor labs (bilirubin)	
Impaired	Increases resistance (splanchnic), which may decrease venous flow from the liver, leading to ischemia. Ultimately, may lead to GI bleeding.
Gastric	
Distension	Primarily caused when cuff leak or esophageal intubation
Stress Ulcer	Ensure compliance with bundles to prevent
Renal	
ensure careful monitoring of renal function, fluid balance, etc.	
Acute renal failure ↓ Output ↑ Fluid Retention	Multiple reasons, but decreased CO decreases renal blood flow, inflammatory response of ventilator, and the effect of abnormal ABGs Results in decreased output, fluid retention

Ventilator-Related Infection

Causes	Patient	• Susceptibility due to being immunocompromised (including immunosuppression from steroids, etc.), stressed • Aspiration or micro-aspiration (around cuff of artificial airway)
	Vent	• Any break in circuit/leak that allows pathogens to enter (open suction, BVM, etc.) • Microaspiration around cuff of artificial airway (including cuff leak, cuff design deficiency)
Signs & Symptoms	Patient	Signs of infection: • Cough with abnormal (or worsened) sputum production (amount, color, consistency) • Increased WBC (+ bands), lactate • Fever, diaphoresis • CXR Infiltrates
	Vent	• Worsening compliance • Patient-ventilator asynchrony • Increasing minute ventilation needs to maintain pH

Ventilator Associated Events (VAE)
including ventilator associated pneumonia (VAP)

Ventilator-Associated Condition	VAC	Respiratory deterioration (increase in PEEP of 3+, or FiO$_2$ increase of 0.2 for 2 days) after a period of stability (2+ days)
Infection-Related Ventilator-Associated Complication	IVAC	VAC (above) + abnormal temp (< 36 C or > 38 C) or WBC (≤ 4000 or ≥ 12,000 cells/mm^3)
Possible and Probable VAP	VAP	IVAC with lab/microbiology evidence of respiratory infection Possible: Gram stain evidence of purulent secretions (or pathogenic pulmonary culture) Probable: Gram stain evidence + growth of a pathogenic organism, or + test for certain viruses, etc.
Ventilated Hospital-Acquired Pneumonia	VHAP	Pneumonia that occurs in patients hospitalized for 2+ days who show signs of infection before intubation

Effects

VAE Bundle*

Main goals include minimizing unnecessary time with an artificial airway and on a ventilator, and using strategies to decrease pathogen transference or growth in the lower respiratory system.

VAE Bundle Item	Rationale
Head of bed at 30-45°	Prevents reflux/aspiration
Avoid NG tubes, use OG tube if necessary	Reduce sinus infections Reduce fluids up esophagus
Oral care with chlorhexidine	Reduce pathogens that might travel into the lungs
Protective cover for tonsillar suction when not in use	Reduce pathogens that might travel into oropharynx
Daily spontaneous breathing trial	Reduce ventilator time
Daily sedation interruption	Reduce ventilator time
Use of specially designed ET tubes and assisted devices	Reduce secretions pooled on the airway cuff
Consider silver-coated ET tube, tapered cuff, or polyurethane material	Reduce microbes in biofilm in the ET tube lumen
Automated cuff pressure monitoring/management	Reduce aspiration/microaspiration around cuff
Use closed suction catheter with vent circuit	Reduce circuit disconnect which can cause sudden PEEP loss
Consider use of HME	Avoid pathogen growth
Perform hand hygiene before and after contact with vent	Avoid pathogen transference

*Summarized in part from: Kallet R. Ventilator bundles in transition: from prevention of ventilator-associated pneumonia to prevention of ventilator-associated events. *Respiratory Care* 2019;64(8):994-1006.

Effects

11 Weaning and Discontinuation

Weaning/Discontinuation Algorithm	11-2
Basic Definitions	11-4
General Strategies	11-5
Assessment for Weaning/Discontinuation	11-6
Vital Signs	11-6
Oxygenation	11-7
Ventilation	11-7
Mechanics	11-8
Integrated Indices	11-8
Acid-Base Balance	11-9
Airway	11-10
Chest Imaging	11-11
Ventilator Muscle/Strength	11-11
Ventilator Drive/Demand	11-11
Cardiovascular	11-12
Electrolytes	11-13
Metabolic	11-13
Nutritional	11-13
Neurological	11-14
Pharmacological	11-15
Renal	11-15
Psychological	11-16
Miscellaneous	11-17
Procedural	11-17
Summarized Indications of Failure	11-18
Rapid Shallow Breathing Index (RSBI)	11-19
Cuff Leak Test	11-20
Extubation Procedure	11-21
Post-Extubation Care	11-22
Reintubation Criteria	11-23
Weaning and Discontinuation Summarized Guidelines	11-24

WEANING

Weaning   11-1

Weaning

Full Support Ventilation

- Ensure optimization and patient-ventilator synchrony
- Has reason for initiation improved or reversed?

Success ↓

Wean Ventilator Settings

- Wean FiO_2 to safe levels
- Consider transition of full support (ventilator breaths) to spontaneous breaths (with support)

Success ↓ *Failure* →

Daily Sedation Interruption

- Goals include minimizing sedation and reducing the duration of mechanical ventilation
- Adequate pain control remains a priority during the sedation interruption
- Sedation is stopped until patient is awake or noted to be agitated/uncomfortable

Failure →

Spontaneous Breathing Trial (SBT) (pg 11-5)

- Coordinated with daily sedation interruption
- Duration recommendations vary: 30 minutes is typical but extended to as long as 120 minutes
- At end of SBT period, evaluate patient (see discontinuation assessment on following pages). There is no single definitive parameter

Failure →

Success ↓

Weaning Parameters (pg 11-6)

- Perform weaning parameters (this is usually a selection of options: VC, NIF (PIMax), RSBI, etc.

Failure →

Discontinuation (Liberation)

Weaning Parameters Met
(see previous page)

↓

Discontinuation
See Discontinuation Assessments, following pages. Note that assessment takes place with the SBT as well. ET Tube: extubation (see pg 11-21) Tracheostomy: maintain airway during initial discontinuation If weaning parameters are borderline and decision made to discontinue ventilator -or- underlying pathophysiology with concerns, consider a bridge therapy: • HFOT (HFNC) • NPPV Then, wean from bridge therapy (see pg 8-12) Monitor closely after discontinuation (perform initial assessment, then reassess at short intervals until stable at baseline)

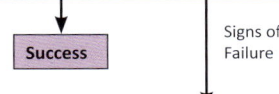

↓ Signs of Failure

Discontinuation Failure?
If patient shows increased WOB, other signs of respiratory distress (vital signs, etc.), consider options: • Initiate and/or increase bridge therapy support • SABA administration (wheezing) • Racemic Epi, heliox, cool aerosol (post-extubation stridor) • Airway clearance (cough, coarse crackles) **If poor mental status, severe distress, inability to show improvement with bridge therapies, consider need to reintubate (preference is for planned reintubation versus emergent reintubation)**

Basic Definitions

Weaning	The reduction of ventilator support and its replacement with spontaneous ventilation.
Spontaneous Breathing Trial (SBT)	The patient is placed on minimal spontaneous settings (often PSV 5/5 or CPAP 5) or on a T-piece and monitored for 30 minutes (or longer if deemed necessary).
Liberation	The ability to breathe without the assistance of the ventilator
Discontinuation	Removal from the ventilator (with the intention of being permanent)
Extubation	The removal of the endotracheal tube, usually occurs with discontinuation
Decannulation	The removal of the tracheostomy tube, often delayed post-discontinuation
Discontinuation failure	The clinical determination that a patient is failing removal from the ventilator. The need to either reinitiate the ventilator (including reintubation if no trach) or initiate rescue therapies (NPPV, HFNC, etc.) is evident.
Difficult-to-Wean	Patients who fail the initial SBT, then require up to 3 SBTs (or 7 days) to pass
Prolonged Wean	Patients who fail 3+ SBTs over more than 7 days (often indicates need for a tracheostomy)
Prolonged Mechanical Ventilation	> 21 days of mechanical ventilation for at least 6-hours/day*

*U.S. Centers for Medicaire and Medicaid Services

General Strategies for Weaning

Note that protocol-driven weaning and discontinuation has been demonstrated to be advantageous in decreasing delays on the ventilator* and that sedation liberation protocols be utilized to minimize sedation to prevent unnecessary delays in liberation.*

Spontaneous Breathing Trial (SBT)	Preferred method in patients intubated > 24 hours: Patient is placed on a spontaneous mode with some sort of pressure augmentation (5-8 cm H_2O) for a period of 30-120 min* Less preferred: use of a T-piece (no support) or CPAP*
SIMV Rate Wean	Place patient on SIMV (volume or pressure) Decrease the mandatory (ventilator) breaths as tolerated, requiring the patient to assume more of the responsibility for the minute volume. Discontinue when the patient can maintain for 1-2 hours at a rate of 4 breaths/minute.
Pressure Support Wean	Patient is placed on PSV (see PSV page 3-16 for initiation details), then the pressure support level is weaned gradually (~1-2 cmH_2O every 2-4 hours)

*ATS/ACCP Clinical Practice Guideline: Liberation from Mechanical Ventilation in Critically Ill Adults. 2017 Update

Assessments for Weaning and Discontinuation Readiness

The following pages present a fairly in-depth guide to assessments used at various points of the weaning and discontinuation process. Not all parameters are used and no one parameter (or even set of parameters) is definitive in making a decision on weaning success or discontinuation readiness

The decision to discontinue invasive ventilation needs to balance the importance of minimizing time on the ventilator with minimizing the risks associated with the need to reintubate.

Intubated Patients: Discontinuing means extubating, with the major risk being the need to reintubate (which increases the risk of aspiration, trauma, or a major event like a code). This requires clinicians to be relatively conservative in making a decision to extubate.

Tracheostomy Patients: Discontinuing means disconnecting the ventilator, but the artificial airway remains. The risks are less here, suggesting clinicians can be more aggressive in attempting to liberate from the ventilator.

> **Resolution of the acute phase of the cause is an important indicator of readiness for discontinuation.**

Vital Signs

Parameter	RR	HR	BP	Temp
Desired Value	stable no significant tachypnea/ bradypnea	stable no significant tachycardia/ bradycardia	stable with no/minimal pressors	within normal range

Respiratory Assessment
See also Chapter 4 for
Patient-Ventilator Assessment and Troubleshooting

Predictive Indices (see chapter 6 for Equations)
Unless otherwise indicated these indices assume minimal ventilator support with spontaneous effort

Oxygenation

Parameter	Desired/Threshold Value
$PaO_2 \leq 0.4\text{-}0.5\ FiO_2$	> 60 mmHg
SaO_2 on FiO_2 up to 0.4	> 90%
PaO_2/FiO_2 ratio	> 200
PaO_2/PAO_2	> 0.35
$P(A\text{-}a)O_2$	< 350 mmHg on $FiO_2 = 1.0$
Q_S/Q_T (shunt %)	< 0.2 (20%)
Hgb	> 8-10 g/dL
Low PEEP	< 8 cmH$_2$O

Ventilation

Parameter	Desired/Threshold Value
$PaCO_2$	< 50 mmHg
$\dot{V}_E$ (spont.)	< 10 to 15 L/min
V_D/V_T	< 0.6
V_T (Spontaneous)	> 5 mL/kg IBW
Respiratory rate (spont.)	< 35/min or > 6-10/min
Respiratory pattern	Regular (or baseline)

Mechanics

Parameter	Desired/Threshold Value
P_{IMAX} (MIF, MIP, NIF)	more negative than -20 to -30 cmH$_2$O
VC	> 10 - 15 mL/kg
MVV	$\geq$ 2 x spontaneous $\dot{V}_E$ (resting) or > 20 L/min
C_{dyn}	$\geq$ 22 mL/cmH$_2$O
C_{stat}	$\geq$ 33 mL/cmH$_2$O
$P_{0.1}$	$\leq$ 6 cmH$_2$O

Integrated Indices

Note that new weaning indices are being investigated regularly. The more common ones are presented here

Parameter	Desired/Threshold Value
RSBI (f/V_T)*	< 100-105 breaths/min/L T-Piece < ~75 on PS or CPAP (see pg 11-19)
SWI (Simplified Weaning Index)	< 9/min > 11/min may indicate failure SWI = [f x (PIP-PEEP)/MIP] x PaCO$_2$/40
CROP index (Compliance, Rate, Oxygenation, and Pressure Index)	> 13 mL/breath/min CROP Index= (Cdyn x MIP x PaO$_2$/PAO$_2$)/f
$P_{0.1}/P_{IMAX}$	< 0.9

Acid-Base Balance

Acid-base should be at baseline or improving towards baseline. Note that any specific metabolic acidosis will increase need for respiratory compensation and risk tiring out the extubated patient.

Imbalance	Acute Causes	Effects
Respiratory Acidosis	Hypoventilation	↑ ventilatory demand
Respiratory Alkalosis	Hyperventilation	↓ ventilatory drive ↑ Hgb affinity for O_2
Metabolic Acidosis	Lactic acidosis Ketoacidosis	↑ ventilatory demand Confusion Pulmonary edema Dysrhythmias (severe)
Metabolic Alkalosis	↓ K^+, Cl^- Nasogastric tube Vomiting	↓ ventilatory drive ↑ Hgb affinity for O_2

Airway

Make reasonable effort to ensure airway will be patent upon extubation. If patient was intubated for airway patency issues (edema, secretion management), additional steps should be taken to ensure the underlying issue has resolved.

Assessment	Clinical Findings
Obstruction	Verify via auscultation, CXR, etc. that there is no acute obstruction (anatomic, bronchospasm, etc.)
Gag Reflex	This can often be noted during routine oral care. If not, very gently insert a small FR suction catheter toward the back of the tongue
Airway Patency	Assess the amount of room available around the ET tube (or trach tube) when the cuff is deflated. • Consider performing a cuff leak test (see pg 11-20). Any leak (auscultated, noted in vent graphics, measured on volume control, etc.) can be considered a positive leak test, although some clinical scenarios may indicate the need for a minimal measured leak. • A leak may not be noted if a large airway is in place (even with cuff down, there may be no space)
Secretions	Ensure secretions are manageable (amount, consistency) and that the patient has an adequate cough (measure PImax, see pg 2-8)

Chest Imaging
Relevant chest imaging should be systematically reviewed. Look for signs of improvement (or lack of). In general, acute processes should be resolved or improving.

Ventilatory Muscles/Strength

> **Bedside Assessment:** Ask patient to hold their head up off the pillow for about 10 seconds. This indicates adequate strength and confirms the ability to follow instruction

Major causes of concern with strength include patient being deconditioned from prolonged ventilator support. This can best be addressed proactively by using early mobility strategies, aggressive weaning, etc. Other concerns include decreased capacity (drugs, malnutrition, sleep deprivation, etc.) and increased load (small ET Tube, ↓ compliance, chest wall restrictions such as obesity)

Ventilatory Drive and Demand

Factors that ↑ Ventilatory Drive	Factors that ↓ Ventilatory Drive
• Acidosis • Agitation • Anxiety • Closed head injury • Drugs (stimulants) • Dyspnea • Fear • Hypoxia • Pain	• Alkalosis • CNS injury or disease • Drugs (depressants) • Electrolyte imbalance • Fatigue • ↓ metabolism • Sedation

Factors that increase Ventilatory Demand:
- ↑ Ventilatory drive (see above)
- ↑ $\dot{V}_{CO_2}$ (See Metabolic Assessment)
- ↑ V_D: Anatomical, mechanical

Cardiovascular Assessment

If on cardiac support of some type, should be stable with reasonable expectation of ventilator discontinuation success.

Parameter	Desired/Threshold Value
ECG	On monitor, should be at baseline and stable (no dysrhythmias)
Stable BP	Stable with minimal hemodynamic supports needed
Fluid Balance	If patient is considerably fluid overloaded, consider diuresing prior to liberation
Anemia	Verify hemoglobin, hematocrit are both acceptable
Hemo Stability	Verify adequate CO, no shock, adeq. LV function, contractility, stable ECG

Electrolyte Assessment

Parameter	Normal Range	Significance
Phosphate (PO_4)	1.4 - 2.7 mg/dL	Decreases in values may indicate a diminished ventilatory drive (interpret in context of patient assessment)
Potassium (K^+)	3.5 - 5.0 mEq/L	
Magnesium (Mg^+)	1.3 - 2.5 mEq/L	

Metabolic Assessment

↑ Metabolism (↑ $\dot{V}_{CO_2}$)	↓ Metabolism (↓ $\dot{V}_{CO_2}$)
• Agitation • Excessive caloric intake (see below) • Fever • Seizures or shivering • Sepsis • Increased WOB	• Malnutrition • Starvation (↓ ventilatory drive and muscles)

Nutritional Assessment

Undernourished	Overnourished
• Resp Muscle atrophy • Pulmonary embolus risk • Pneumonia/infection risk	• ↑ CO_2 production (may worsen weaning outcomes) • ↑ WOB • ↑ $\dot{V}E$ requirement

Appropriate caloric intake
- Appropriate nutrition-caloric intake (~25-30 kcal/kg):
  1.5 - 2 x REE (resting energy expenditure)
- Appropriate protein intake: 1-1.5 gm/kg/day

Neurologic Assessment

A specific neuro assessment should be considered if an underlying neuro concern. As with other assessments, information should be viewed against the patient's baseline, expectation to recover, etc.

Parameter	Desired/Threshold Value
Intracranial Pressure (ICP)	< 20 mmHg see page 9-41
Cerebral Perfusing Pressure (CPP)	60-80 mmHg see page 9-38
Seizure Activity	Seizures should be at baseline, or controlled if acute cause
Neural Drive to Breathe	see Ventilator Drive, pg 11-11
Mental Status	Should be at baseline See other causes in Psych Assessment (page 11-16)

Pharmacological Assessment

Drugs should be assessed for their impact on drive to breathe and mental status

Drug Type	Potential Effects
• Hypnotics • Sedatives • Narcotics • Tranquilizers	↓ Ventilatory drive and/or mental response
• Stimulants	↑ Ventilatory drive
• Aminoglycosides (potentates NMBAs) • Corticosteroids • Muscle Relaxants • Neuromuscular blockers*	↓ Ventilatory muscle function

* NMBAs are an absolute contraindication to discontinuing full ventilatory support

Renal Assessment

Renal Factors	Comments
Acid-base abnormalities	Affects drive and load
Fluid imbalance Intake & Output Renal Insufficiency	Overload impairs pulmonary gas exchange and leads to pulmonary edema (Adequate output > 1000 mL/day and equal to intake)
Electrolyte imbalance	Causes ventilatory muscle weakness

Psychological Assessment

There are many psychological factors to consider, some predictable and others not. This list is not exhaustive, but looks at some of the most common considerations:

Factor	Considerations
Anxiety/Fear	• Communicate clearly with patient • Have familiar people at bedside • Consider anti-anxiety drugs
Combativeness	• Consider change in sedation • Accelerate extubation if clinically acceptable (combativeness may be related to fear/claustrophobia)
Delirium	• Consider pharmacological intervention
Pain	• Ask patient about pain, if able or • Manage pain by watching for patient cues (grimacing, etc.) and vitals
Psychological Dependence on Ventilator	• Use slow wean strategy - small steps
Sleep Deprivation	• Ensure patient-ventilator synchrony • Create environment that mimics day/night (minimize as many pt care interactions as possible at night, keep noise to a minimum at night) • Consider sleep aids (eye mask, earplugs, white noise)
Withdrawal (drugs, alcohol)	• Consider with team: may require pharmacologic treatment • Patient may need to remain intubated until acute withdrawal symptoms have passed

Miscellaneous Factors
- Note underlying activity tolerance
- Assess and optimize patient positioning (usually preference is for being upright in a sitting position)
- Note presence of underlying pathophysiologies (baseline)
- Asses for other systems (gastrointestinal including ascites, hyperglycemia, sepsis/infection, kidney/metabolic, etc.)
- Consider need for impending surgical procedures requiring general anesthetics, especially with trauma (avoid discontinuing if the patient has a planned need for reintubation in the near future)

Procedural factors

- **Weaning Procedures Used**
    - Time of day (avoid evenings, nights, and shift change)
    - Interruptions, disruptions (tests, for example)
    - Excessive time of wean (SBT > 120 min, for example)

- **Technical Factors**
    - Insufficient settings (PS level, PEEP, trigger sensitivity)
    - Insufficient method/mode (intolerance of SIMV wean, etc.)

Summarized Indicators of Weaning Failure

Monitor	Signs of Failure
Respiratory *assessment that indicates distress, tiring*	
RR	> 30 - 35 breaths/min or < 10 breaths/min or > 50% change
V_T	< 5 mL/kg (< 250 mL in adults)
↑ WOB	↑ Accessory muscle use Paradoxical Breathing
RSBI*	> 100-105 breaths/min/L (T-piece) (consider > 75 if by CPAP or low PS)
ABGs/Oxygenation	
PaO_2	< 50-60 mmHg
SaO_2	< 85-90%
$PaCO_2$	↑ 10+ mmHg from baseline
pH	↓ 0.10+ from baseline or < 7.30
Cardiovascular	
HR	Change by 20% or < 60/min or > 120 - 140/min
BP	Change > 20% systolic or 10% diastolic or < 90 mmHg or > 180 mmHg systolic > 90 mmHg diastolic
ECG	Significant arrhythmias, angina, ↑ PAWP
Other	
Mental Status	Agitation, anxiety, coma, somnolence
Pain/Discomfort	Inability to manage pain
Secretions	Inability to manage

*For common causes of discontinuation failure, refer to the assessment throughout this chapter

Rapid Shallow Breathing Index (RSBI)

Many ventilators automatically calculate an RSBI. The value obtained is dependent on how the RSBI is performed, with a lower (better) RSBI more likely when PSV or CPAP are used (versus a T-piece trial).

Performing RSBI on Minimal PSV or CPAP (Common)
- Ensure patient is on reasonably low settings:
  - Spontaneous mode (typically PSV or CPAP)
  - Baseline PEEP (~5 cmH$_2$O)
  - Minimal or no pressure support/ATC
- If performing on higher settings, consider carefully in context of other weaning parameters (RSBI is not meant to be the single determinant of readiness to discontinue support)
- Some evidence recommends using a lower threshold (prediction of discontinuation success = < 75 breaths/min/L) when using CPAP or PSV on a ventilator*

Performing RSBI on a T-Piece (Uncommon)
1. Remove the patient from the ventilator (place on T-piece)
2. Allow enough time for spontaneous breathing pattern to stabilize
3. Measure expired $\dot{V}_E$ and RR for one minute with respirometer Divide $\dot{V}_E$ by frequency f to obtain average V_T
4. Divide f by V_T to obtain RSBI (f / V_T)
5. Typically a value of < 105 is used to predict success, although some studies suggest < 100 as more predictive

Consider RSBI in Context of Clinical State:*
- COPD: may not be appropriate
- Cardiac: consider lowest PEEP or CPAP (PEEP may disguise underlying dysfunction - see page 9-22)
- Neurosurgical: may not be appropriate (mental status is a greater determinant than lung function)
- Prolonged Weans: consider the value of trending RSBI versus use of a specific value
- Noninvasive Ventilation: RSBI has been shown to have value in predicting successful weaning (> 105 may indicate need to intubate)

*Karthika M, Enezi F, Pillai L, Arabi Y. Rapid shallow breathing index. Ann Thoracic Med. 2016 Jul-Sep:11(3);167-176.

Cuff Leak Test

A lack of a cuff leak (upper airway) may indicate a higher risk for post-extubation stridor

- Cuff leak test should be considered for patients at high risk for post-extubation stridor*
  - A passed test indicates air flow around the ET tube and is considered definitive (meaning the anatomic airway is patent)
  - A failed test has no air flow around the ET tube. The results should be evaluated in context (ET tube size, airway abnormalities, etc.). Then, consider administration of systemic steroids 4+ hrs before extubating (there's no need to repeat the cuff leak test after this).*

*ATS/ACCP Clinical Practice Guideline: Liberation from Mechanical Ventilation in Critically Ill Adults. 2017 Update

Quantitative (Measured) Cuff Leak Test

1. Place patient on full support mode (A/C)
2. Suction above the cuff (oral suction) and below the cuff (suction catheter via ET tube)
3. With cuff inflated: note inspiratory (V_{TI}) and expiratory (V_{TE}) tidal volumes
4. Deflate the cuff and note the average V_{TI} and V_{TE} over several breaths
5. Reinflate the cuff and return ventilator to previous settings.
6. Subtract the average V_{TE} (cuff deflated) from the V_{TI} (cuff inflated). This is the leak.

Qualitative (Observed) Cuff Leak Test

1. Place patient on full support mode (A/C)
2. Suction above the cuff (oral suction) and below the cuff (suction catheter via ET tube)
3. Deflate cuff while watching ventilator graphics (observe for a leak, see page 5-46) while auscultating over throat (listen for an audible leak).

Extubation Procedure

Equipment Needed:
- Manual resuscitation bag with reservoir for 100% F_iO_2 with mask
- Oxygen source
- Oxygen mask or cannula (hooked up and running)
- High-volume suction source and equipment (appropriately sized catheter, large bore oral suction device)
- Oral and pharyngeal airways
- Reintubation equipment (if needed)
- A 10 cc syringe (for cuff deflation)
- Disposable towel/pad

Procedure:
- Choose an appropriate time of the day (preferably AM) and not during shift change.
- Explain the procedure to the patient.
- Consider removal of NG/OG tube simultaneously with ET tube.
- Monitor patient throughout and after procedure (ECG, SpO_2).
- Sit patient in semi- or high Fowler's position.
- Pre-oxygenate patient with 100% F_iO_2.
- Suction the mouth and pharynx.
- Give large breath with hold as the cuff is being deflated to force secretions above the cuff (repeat until clear).
- Loosen the tape or ET Tube holder.
- Instruct patient to cough as ET tube is being removed (or hyper inflate patient).
- Remove tube (including OG/NG if appropriate) quickly and smoothly as pt. coughs.
- Instruct the patient to cough directly after the ET tube is removed.
- Have patient speak a word or two.
- Administer the same (or slightly higher) F_iO_2 as prior to extubation.
- Auscultate for breath sounds, auscultate throat for stridor
- Encourage the patient to take deep breaths and cough.
- Monitor the patient closely.

Post-Extubation Care

Patients should be assessed immediately following extubation, both initially and then periodically (at least several times). Systematic assessment should include:

- Direct patient to cough
- Direct patient to say a few words
  (verifies mental status, vocal cord function)
- Auscultate (lung fields and throat)
- Check vital signs (HR, RR, BP, SpO_2)
- Check WOB (accessory muscles, paradoxical breathing, diaphoresis)

If stridor is present, consider:
- Cool aerosol by mask (supplemental O_2 as needed)
- Nebulized racemic epinephrine (2-3 unit dosages may be necessary)
- Heliox (80/20 or 70/30) delivered via nonrebreather
- Concurrent systemic steroid administration
- If stridor is accompanied by diminished breath sounds and significant WOB, consider immediate reintubation

Reintubation Criteria

Making the decision to reintubate ranges from being clear (severe distress, inability to protect airway) to unclear (slowly diminishing function, secretion management issues)

HR	Clinically significant tachycardia (urgent) or bradycardia (often emergent)
RR	Clinically significant tachypnea (with tiring) or bradypnea
$\dot{V}_E$	An increased minute ventilation is associated with the need to reintubate
BP	Clinically significant hypertension or hypotension (especially low diastolic pressure)
ECG	Abnormal rhythms, especially if new or symptomatic
P/F	Worsening P/F or S/F ratio

Consider also:

Mental Status	Worsening, unable to follow commands (versus baseline)
Secretions	Ability to manage own secretions with or without reasonable adjuncts (including type of adjunct, suctioning frequency, etc.)
Airway Patency	If airway is not patent (stridor that is significantly affecting oxygen or ventilation), reestablish the airway
SBT History	Greater failed SBTs (with or without failed extubations) may indicate a need to consider reintubation more aggressively
Prognosis	Consider likelihood of overall recovery and the appropriateness of palliative measures per patient's wishes

Weaning

Weaning and Discontinuation Summarized Guidelines
adapted in part from ACCP/AARC/ACCCM Evidence-Based Guidelines for Weaning and Discontinuing Ventilator Support

---

On Ventilator for > 24-hours
Search for causes of need for ventilator
Attempt to reverses causes (see pg 11-6)

Assess Readiness for Discontinuation

- Evidence of reversal (at least partially) of underlying cause
- Confirm clinical stability (pH in baseline range)
- Confirm adequate oxygenation (P/F > 150-200, PEEP ≤ 5-8, FiO_2 ≤ 0.4-0.5)
- Confirm hemo stability (no significant hypotension, minimal vasopressors, no ischemia)
- Confirm ability to initiate inspiration

Pass ↓

Place patient on 3-5 minutes of spontaneous breathing
preference for pressure augmentation 5-8 cmH₂O during SBT

Perform discontinuation assessment:
- Acceptable gas exchange
- Oxygenation: SpO_2, PaO_2 acceptable
- Ventilation: $PaCO_2$ stable, pH ≥ 7.32
- Hemo: HR < 120-140 or < 20% change, BP stable with minimal pressors
- Stable ventilator pattern (RR < 30-35 for most)
- Assess mental status, discomfort/pain, diaphoresis, WOB

Pass ↓   Fail ↓

↓ Pass

Continue SBT for 30-120 min

Assess patient tolerance (see pg 11-8) → Fail

↓ Pass

Consider for Discontinuation

Assess underlying airway patency
Assess ability to protect own airway
Perform cuff leak test if high-risk (see pg 11-20) → Fail

↓ Pass

Extubate

Fail →

Place patient on a stable, nonfatiguing, comfortable form of ventilatory support

Explore and correct causes of failure (see pg 11-6)
Ensure the following minimum criteria:
- Adequate oxygenation ($PaO_2 \geq 60$ on $FIO_2 \leq 0.4$ and PEEP $\leq 5-8$; P/F $\geq 150-200$)
- Adequate acid-base: $PaCO_2$ stable, pH ≥ 7.32
- Hemo stability (HR < 140, stable BP, minimal pressors)
- Afebrile
- Adequate mental status (GCS, no significant sedation)
- Adequate cough
- Resolution of acute phase of illness/disease (or discontinuation success looks possible)

Difficult to Wean: Gradual Discontinuation

- Slow-paced approach. Once at about 50% support, consider gradual lengthening of self-breathing trials
- Consider need for tracheostomy placement

*MacIntyre N, Cook D, Ely E, Epstein S, Fink F, Heffner J, Hess D, Hubmayer R, Scheinhorn D. Evidence-based guidelines for weaning and discontinuing ventilator support: a collective task force facilitated by the American College of Chest Physicians; the American Association for Respiratory Care, and the American College of Critical Care Medicine. Chest 2001;120(6 suppl):375S-395S. with updates in 2017 (ATS/ACCP)

A Appendix

Basic Units of Measure A-2
Gas Phase Symbols A-2
Blood Phase Symbols A-2
Conversions
   Metric A-3
   U.S./Metric Equivalents A-3
   Temperature (C ↔ F) A-4
   Weight (kg ↔ lb) A-4
   Height (ft ↔ in ↔ cm) A-4
Abbreviations A-5
Evidence-Based Guidelines (AARC) A-7

Basic Units of Measure

cm H$_2$O	centimeters of water pressure
gm%	gram percent (number of grams per 100 grams of total weight)
kg	kilograms
kPa	kiloPascals (SI unit for pressure)
mg	milligrams
mL	milliliters
mm Hg	millimeters of mercury (pressure)
vol%	volume percent (number of mL in a substance per 100 mL of volume)
L/min	liters per minute
mEq/L	milliequivalents per liter
torr	unit of measure roughly equivalent to mm Hg

Gas Phase Symbols

D	Diffusion
F	Fractional concentration of a gas
P	Partial pressure of a gas
$\bar{P}$	Mean pressure of a gas
R	Respiratory exchange ratio
V	Volume of a gas
$\dot{V}$	Flow of a gas (volume/time)

Blood Phase Symbols

Q	Volume of blood
$\dot{Q}$	Blood flow (cardiac output) in L/min
C	Concentration (content in the blood phase)
S	Saturation in the blood phase

Conversions

Metric Measures

Linear		Weight		Volume	
kilometer (km)	m × 10^3	kilogram (kg)	g × 10^3	kiloliter	L × 10^3
decameter	m × 10	decagram	g × 10	decaliter	L × 10
meter (m)		gram (g)		liter (L)	
decimeter	m × 10^{-1}	decigram	g × 10^{-1}	deciliter (dL)	L × 10^{-1}
centimeter (cm)	m × 10^{-2}	centigram	g × 10^{-2}	centiliter	L × 10^{-2}
millimeter (mm)	m × 10^{-3}	milligram (mg)	g × 10^{-3}	milliliter (mL)	L × 10^{-3}
micrometer (µ)	m × 10^{-6}	microgram (µg)	g × 10^{-6}	microliter (µL)	L × 10^{-6}

U.S. Customary and Metric Equivalents

1 inch	2.54 cm	1 ounce (oz)	28.35 g	1 ounce (fl)	29.57 mL
1 foot	.0348 m	1 pound	454 g	1 quart	0.9463 L
1 mile	1.609 km	1 gram	0.0352 oz	1 gallon	3.785 L
1 micron	3.937 × 10^{-5} in	1 kilogram	2.2 lb	cubic inch (in^3)	16.39 mL
1 centimeter	0.3937 in			cubic foot (ft^3)	28.32 L
1 meter	39.37 in			1 liter	1.057 qt

Temperature

°C = (°F-32) x 5/9	
°F = (°C x 9/5) + 32	
°F	°C
32	0
90	32.2
91	32.8
92	33.3
93	33.4
94	34.4
95	35.0
96	35.6
97	36.1
98	36.7
98.6	37.0
99	37.2
100	37.8
101	38.3
102	38.9
103	39.4
104	40.0
105	40.6
106	41.1
107	41.7
108	42.2
109	42.8

While 37 C is generally seen as "perfect normal" a range of normals is more appropriate

Height

1 Foot = 12 inches		
1 inch = 2.54 centimeters		
Ft	in.	cm.
5' 0"	60	152.4
5' 1"	61	154.9
5' 2"	62	157.5
5' 3"	63	160.0
5' 4"	64	162.6
5' 5"	65	165.1
5' 6"	66	167.6
5' 7"	67	170.2
5' 8"	68	172.7
5' 9"	69	175.3
5' 10"	70	177.8
5' 11"	71	180.3
6' 0"	72	182.9
6' 1"	73	185.4
6' 2"	74	188.0
6' 3"	75	190.5
6' 4"	76	193.0
6' 5"	77	195.6
6' 6"	78	198.1
6' 7"	79	200.7
6' 8"	80	203.2
6' 9"	81	205.7

Weight

1 kilogram = 2.2 pounds					
kg	lb	kg	lb	kg	lb
1	2.2	10	22.0	90	198.4
2	4.4	20	44.0	100	220.5
3	6.6	30	66.0	110	242.5
4	8.8	40	88.0	120	264.6
5	11.0	50	110.0	130	286.6
6	13.2	60	132.0	140	308.6
7	15.4	70	154.0	150	330.7
8	17.6	80	176.0	160	352.7

Abbreviations

Abbreviation	Definition
ΔP	Delta-P (change pressure) Driving pressure
AARC	American Association of Respiratory Care
A/C	Assist/control
ACCP	American College of Chest Physicians
ADH	Anti-diuretic hormone
ABG	Arterial blood gas
APRV	Airway pressure release ventilation
APV	Adaptive pressure ventilation
ARDS	Adult respiratory distress syndrome
ASV	Adaptive support ventilation
ATC	Automatic tube compensation
BiPAP	Bi-level positive airway pressure
BP	Blood pressure
BPdia	Diastolic blood pressure
BPsys	Systolic blood pressure
B-P	Broncho-pleural
BSA	Body surface area
CABG	Coronary artery bypass graft
CaO_2	Arterial oxygen content
$Ca-\overline{v}O_2$	Arterial–mixed venous O_2 content difference
Ccw	Compliance of the chest wall
Cdyn	Dynamic compliance
CF	Conversion factor
CI	Cardiac index
CL	Compliance of the lung
CLT	Compliance of the lung and thorax
cmH_2O	Centimeters of water
CNS	Central nervous system
CO	Cardiac output
CO	Carbon monoxide
CO_2	Carbon dioxide
COPD	Chronic obstructive pulmonary disease
CPAP	Continuous positive airway pressure
CPP	Cerebral perfusion pressure
Cstat	Static compliance
Ctubing	Compliance of the tubing
CV	Cardiovascular
CVA	Cerebrovascular accident
CVP	Central venous pressure
CXR	Chest x-ray
DP	Driving Pressure
ECG	Electrocardiogram
ECMO	Extracorporeal membrane oxygenation
EPAP	Expiratory positive airway pressure
et	End-tidal
ET	Endotracheal
f	Frequency (ventilator rate)
FiO_2	Fraction of inspired oxygen
FRC	Functional residual capacity
GI	Gastrointestinal
HFNC	High-flow nasal cannula
HFOT	High-frequency oxygen therapy
Hgb	Hemoglobin
HME	Heat moisture exchanger
HR	Heart rate
ICP	Intracranial pressure
I:E	Inspiratory/expiratory ratio
IPAP	Inspiratory positive airway pressure
IRV	Inverse ratio ventilation
J	Joule
JVD	Jugular vein distention
kg	Kilogram
LIP	Lower inflection point
LOC	Level of consciousness
LV	Left ventricle
MAP	Mean arterial pressure
mAW	Mean airway pressure
MDI	Metered dose inhaler
MIF	Maximal inspiratory force
MIP	Maximal inspiratory pressure
mmHg	millimeters of mercury
mPAW	Mean airway pressure
MV	Mechanical ventilation
MV	Minute ventilation
NIF	Negative inspiratory force
NIV	Noninvasive ventilation
NPPV	Noninvasive positive pressure ventilation
O_2ER	Oxygen extraction ratio
$PA-aO_2$	Alveolar-arterial oxygen partial pressure difference
$PaCO_2$	Partial pressure of arterial carbon dioxide
P-ACV	Pressure-assist/control ventilation
PAPD	Pulmonary artery diastolic pressure
Palv	Alveolar pressure

PAMP	Pulmonary artery mean pressure
PaO$_2$	Partial pressure of arterial oxygen
PAO$_2$	Partial pressure of alveolar oxygen
PAOP	Pulmonary artery occlusion pressure
PAP	Pulmonary artery pressure
Paug	Pressure augmentation
PAV	Proportional assist ventilation
Paw	Airway pressure
$\overline{Paw}$	Mean airway pressure
Pawo	Pressure at airway opening
PASP	Pulmonary artery systolic pressure
PAWD	Pulmonary artery wedge pressure
PCWP	Pulmonary capillary wedge pressure
PB	Barometric pressure
PBW	Predicted body weight
PEEP	Positive end-expiratory pressure
pH	Negative log of hydrogen ion concentration
PImax	Maximal inspiratory pressure
PIP	Peak inspiratory pressure
P-IRV	Pressure-inverse ratio ventilation
PIT	Intrathoracic pressure
P-MMV	Pressure-mandatory minute ventilation
PMI	Point of maximal impulse
PP	Pulse pressure
Ppl	Intrapleural pressure
Ppeak	Peak inspiratory pressure
Pplat	Inspiratory plateau pressure
PPV	Positive pressure ventilation
PRVC	Pressure regulated volume control
P-SIMV	Pressure-synchronized intermittent mandatory ventilation
PSV	Pressure support ventilation
PtcO$_2$	Transcutaneous partial pressure of oxygen
PV	Pressure ventilation
PVO$_2$	Partial pressure of oxygen in mixed venous blood
PVR	Pulmonary vascular resistance
Qs/Qt	Physiological shunt
Raw	Airway resistance
RHF	Right heart failure
RR	Spontaneous respiratory rate
SaO$_2$	Saturation of arterial oxygen
SCCM	Society of Critical Care Medicine
SpO$_2$	Saturation of arterial oxygen by pulse oximeter
SvO$_2$	Saturation of oxygen in mixed venous blood
SVR	Systemic vascular resistance
TE	Expiratory time
T-E	Tracheo-esophageal
TI	Inspiratory time
Ttot	Total cycle time
UIP	Upper inflection point
UO	Urinary output
V	Volume
$\dot{V}$	Flow
VA	Alveolar volume
$\dot{V}_A$	Alveolar ventilation
V-ACV	Volume-assist/control ventilation
VAPS	Volume assured pressure support
VCO$_2$	Volume of carbon dioxide production
VD	Deadspace volume
$\dot{V}_D$	Deadspace ventilation
VD/VT	Deadspace/tidal volume ratio
$\dot{V}_E$	Minute ventilation
$\dot{V}_{Emech}$	Minute ventilation mechanical
$\dot{V}_{Espont}$	Minute ventilation spontaneous
VILI	Ventilator-induced lung injury
V-IRV	Volume-inverse ratio ventilation
V-MMV	Volume-mandatory minute ventilation
$\dot{V}_{O_2}$	Volume of oxygen consumption
VPC	Variable pressure support
V-P	Volume-pressure (curve)
VS	Volume support
V-SIMV	Volume-synchronized intermittent mandatory ventilation
VT	Tidal volume
Vtubing	Volume loss to tubing
V/Q	Ventilation/perfusion ratio
WOB	Work of breathing
VV	Volume ventilation

Capnography/Capnometry during Mechanical Ventilation[1,2]
(AARC Expert Panel Reference-Based Guideline)

Indications
- Verification of artificial airway placement: All intubations must be confirmed by $PETCO_2$ measurement
- Assessment of pulmonary circulation and respiratory status: may be quicker than pulse oximetry in pts with lung disease, monitors adequacy of pulmonary, systemic, and coronary blood flow, and in screening for a pulmonary emboli
- Optimization of mechanical ventilation: continuous monitoring of ventilator and circuit functional status, helps evaluate efficiency of ventilation, severity of disease, V/Q during independent lung ventilation, and monitoring of inspired CO_2 when therapeutically administered.
- Evaluation of capnogram: May be useful in detecting rebreathing of CO_2, obstructive disease, NMBA, and effectiveness of compressions during CPR.

Contraindications:
None

Hazards / Complications
- Increased deadspace
- May increase weight/strain on artificial airway/circuit/line

Monitoring
- Ventilatory variables: V_T, f, PEEP, I:E, PIP, FIO_2
- Hemodynamic variables: BP (sys & pulm), CO, shunt, V/Q imbalances

Frequency:
PRN, during intubation

Limitations
- Is not a substitute for assessing $PaCO_2$
- Reliability may be affected by: respiratory gas mixture, RR, freon, secretions/condensate, filters, leaks, low cardiac output or V_T

---

[1] Adapted from: AARC Clinical Practice Guideline: Capnography/capnometry during mechanical ventilation; *Respiratory Care:* 56(4)2011
[2] Evaluation of CO_2 in respiratory gases on MV patients

Endotracheal Suctioning of Mechanically Ventilated Adults and Children[1,2]
(AARC Expert Panel Reference-Based Guideline)

Indications
- Maintain airway patency
- Obtain sputum specimen
- Remove accumulated secretions as evidenced by:
  - Coarse crackles over trachea
  - Sawtooth pattern on Flow-Volume Loop
  - ABG deterioration
  - Acute respiratory distress
  - Suspected aspiration
  - Ineffective cough
  - Vent changes (↑ PIP in volume modes, ↓ V_T in pressure modes)
  - Visible secretions in airway
  - Suspected aspiration

Contraindications
Relative: Adverse reaction or worsening clinical condition from the procedure.

Frequency: Only when clinically indicated to maintain airway patency

Hazards/Complications
- Atelectasis
- Bronchospasm/constriction
- Cardiac arrhythmia/arrest
- Hemorrhage/bleeding
- Hypo/hypertension
- Hypoxia/hypoxemia
- ↑ ICP
- Infection (patient or caregiver)
- Interruption of MV
- Mucosal trauma
- Saline instillation may result in:
- Excessive cough, ↓ SaO_2, Bronchospasm, Dislodgement of biofilm, pain, anxiety, dyspnea, tachycardia, ↑ ICP

Monitoring
ABGs/SaO_2, BS, cough effort, CV parameters (BP, HR, EKG), ICP, RR and pattern, skin color, sputum prod (color, volume, consistency, odor), ventilator parameters (PIP, Pplat, VT, graphics, FIO_2).

---

[1] adapted from the AARC Clinical Practice Guideline: Endotracheal Suction of Mechanically Ventilated Adults and Children with Artificial Airways, *Respiratory Care*: 55(6)2010.

[2] A component of bronchial hygiene therapy involving the mechanical aspiration of pulmonary secretions from a patient with an artificial airway.

Humidification during Invasive and Noninvasive Mechanical Ventilation[1]
(AARC Expert Panel Reference-Based Guideline)

Indication
Mandatory when mechanically ventilated, with ET Tube or Tracheostomy, but optional with NPPV

Contraindication
None except HME when:
- Body temperature < 32°C, concurrent aerosol therapy, expired V_T < 70% of delivered V_T, spont $\dot{V}_E$ > 10 L/min, thick, copious, or bloody secretions, with low VT strategies (ARDS, etc.)
- Do not use HME with NPPV with large mask leaks

Monitoring
Check: alarm settings (41°C at highest) (HR), humidifier temp setting (HR), inspired gas temp (37°C at the wye) (HR), water level and feed system (HR), sputum quantity and consistency
Remove condensate in circuit
Replace HMEs contaminated with secretions

Frequency:
Continuous during gas therapy

Hazards/Complications
- Burns (patient or caregiver) (HH)
- Electrical shock (HH)
- Hypo/hyperthermia
- Hypoventilation (HME → ↑VD)
- ↑ Resistive WOB through humidifier
- Infection (nosocomial)
- Tracheal lavage (pooled condensate or overfilling) (HH)
- Underhydration (mucous impaction or plugging of airways → air-trapping, hypoventilation, ↑ WOB
- Ventilator malperformance: pooled condensate → ↑ airway pressures or asynchrony with patient (HH)
- HME → ineffective low pressure alarm during disconnection
- Pt-Vent dyssynchrony due to pooled condensation (HH)

Clinical Goal
Humidified and warmed inspired gases without hazards or complications.

HH = heated humidity, HME = heat moisture exchanger

[1] adapted from AARC Clinical Practice Guideline: Humidification during invasive and noninvasive mechanical ventilation; *Respiratory Care*: 57(5): 2012.

In Hospital Transport of the Mechanically Ventilated Patient [1]
(AARC Expert Panel Reference-Based Guideline)

Indications
Following a careful evaluation of the risk-benefit ratio

Contraindications
- All members of transport team are not present..
- *Inability during transport to:* Adequately monitor CV status
- Maintain acceptable hemodynamic performance
- Maintain airway control
- Provide adequate O_2 and ventilation

Monitoring
Same as during stationary care.
Continuous: ECG, HR, BP (if invasive line), SpO_2
Intermittent: BS, RR, BP (no invasive line), PIP, V_T

Hazards/Complications
- Accidental extubation or removal of IV access due to movement
- CV instability
- Equipment failure
- Hyperventilation (manual ventilation)
- Inadvertent disconnection of IVs or MV support
- Loss of O_2 supply
- Loss of PEEP/CPAP
- Position changes causing $\downarrow$ BP, $\downarrow$ PaO_2, and/or $\uparrow$ $PaCO_2$
- VAP

Assessment of Need: Risk versus benefit

Assessment of Outcome: Safe arrival

Infection Control: Universal Precautions, disinfection of equip between patients, CDC recommendations for TB risk.

[1] adapted from AARC Clinical Practice Guideline: In-Hospital transport of the mechanically ventilated patient; *Respiratory Care*: 47(6):2002.

Removal of the Endotracheal Tube - 2007[1]
(AARC Expert Panel Reference-Based Guideline)

Indications
- Airway control no longer necessary and patient is able to maintain patent airway and adequate spontaneous ventilation (i.e. adequate neuro drive, muscle strength, cough)
- Artificial airway obstruction (not able to be cleared rapidly)
- Discontinuance of further medical care

Contraindications:
No absolute

Hazards/Complications
- **Hypoxemia** (aspiration, atelectasis, bronchospasm, hypoventilation, laryngospasm, low O_2, pulmonary edema)
- **Hypercapnia** (bronchospasm, excessive WOB, muscle weakness, upper airway edema)
- **Death** (discontinuance of medical care)

Assessment of Readiness
Artificial airway no longer needed as indicated by reversal of cause, adequate spontaneous ventilation and meet readiness criteria:

- ***Maintain adequate PaO_2:*** $PaO_2/F_iO_2 > 150\text{-}200$,
- $PEEP \leq 5\text{-}8$ cm H_2O and
- $FIO_2 \leq 0.4\text{-}0.5$
- Maintain appropriate pH > 7.25 and $PaCO_2$
- $C_{thorax} > 25$ mL/cmH_2O
- $f < 35$/min (adult)
- Modified CROP $\geq 0.1\text{-}0.15$ mL.mmHg/breaths/min/mL/kg
- MVV > $2 \times \dot{V}_E$ (resting)
- NIP > - 20-30 cm H_2O
- O_2 cost of breathing < 15% total
- $P.0.1 < 6$ cm H_2O
- $PEF \geq 60$ L/min
- RSBI ≤ 105 (modified RSBI $\leq$ 8-11 breaths/min.mL.kg)
- SMIP > 57.5
- Successful SBT (30-120 min) with low CPAP (5 cmH_2O) or low PS (5-7 cmH_2O) (i.e., adequate respiratory pattern, gas exchange, hemo stability and comfort)
- VC > 10 mL/kg (ideal)
- $V_D/V_T < 0.6$
- $\dot{V}_E$ (spont) < 10 L/min
- WOB < 0.8 J/L.

(continued from previous page)	
Assessment of Outcome/ Monitoring Assess/monitor: ABGs, adequate spontaneous ventilation & oxygenation, airway patency, chest x-ray, complications, hemodynamics, neuro status, VS, WOB Note: Attentive monitoring, prompt identification of respiratory distress and maintaining patent airway is essential. **Infection Control** Follow CDC Standard Precautions	**Resolution of need for airway protection:** Adequate airway protective reflexes Easily managed secretions Normal consciousness **Other Considerations** Electrolytes Hemodynamics Nutrition Prophylactic meds (lidocaine, steroids) Reintubation need Risk factors Upper airway obstruction/ edema

[1] Adapted from AARC Clinical Practice Guideline: Removal of the Endotracheal Tube – 2007 Revision & Update; *Respiratory Care*: 52(1)2007.

Index

A

A-aDO$_2$ 6-4
AARC Guidelines
 Capnography/Capnometry during Mechanical Ventilation A-7
 Endotracheal Suctioning of Mechanically Ventilated Adults and Children A-8
 Humidification During Mechanical Ventilation 7-43, A-9
 In Hospital Transport of the Mechanically Ventilated Patient A-10
 Removal of the Endotracheal Tube A-11
 Tracheostomy Care (Adults) 7-9
Abbreviations
 basic units of measure A-2
 blood phase symbols A-2
 gas phase symbols A-2
ABG. See Acid-Base
ACCP/AARC/ACCCM Guidelines (Weaning) 11-24

Acid-Base
 and ARF 1-4
 and weaning 11-9
 equations 6-2
 management 7-16–7-19
 values 4-9
ACPE. See Congestive Heart Failure
Acute Respiratory Distress Syndrome 9-2–9-10
 acid-base targets 9-7
 ARDSnet 9-8–9-9
 assessment 9-3
 Berlin definition 9-3
 diagnosis 9-3
 etiology 9-2
 FiO$_2$/PEEP tables 9-8
 management 9-7
 pathophysiology 9-4
 weaning 9-7, 9-10
Acute Respiratory Failure 1-2
 noninvasive algorithm 8-8
 parameters 1-8
 types 1-4
Adaptive Pressure Ventilation (APV) 3-31. See also Pressure Regulated

Volume Control
Adaptive Support Ventilation (ASV) 3-37
Air-hunger 5-48
Air-trapping. See auto PEEP
Airway
 adjuncts 7-3
 assessment 7-4
 management 7-2
 patency 4-4
 weaning assessment 11-10
Airway Clearance 7-37
Airway Obstruction 1-5, 10-2
 adjuncts 7-3
 strategies 10-2
Airway Oscillations 7-39
Airway Pressure Release Ventilation (APRV) 3-20–3-25
 improving oxygenation 3-23
 improving ventilation 3-24
 initial rescue settings 3-21
 pressure support use 3-22
 weaning 3-25
Airway Pressures. See Mean Airway Pressure
Airway Resistance (Raw) 4-12

changes in 4-14
equation 6-19
Alarms 2-23
problems 2-23
setting 2-23
Alveolar
ventilation 6-12
volume 6-12
Alveolar Air Equation 6-4
Analgesia 7-18
and weaning 11-2
Anatomical Vd/Vt Ratio 6-13
Anion Gap 6-2
Apnea
alarm 2-23
APRV. See Airway Pressure Release Ventilation (APRV)
APV. See Pressure-Regulated Volume Control
ARDS. See Acute Respiratory Distress Syndrome
ARDSnet 9-8
FiO$_2$/PEEP tables 9-8
Arterial/Alveolar O$_2$ Tension 6-5
Arterial-Venous O$_2$ Content Difference 6-5

Artificial Airway 7-4
and proning 7-35
asynchrony 7-45
establishing 7-6
Aspiration
and ARDS 9-2
Assessment 4-6
acid-base 4-9
oxygenation 4-10
patient 4-6
respiratory distress 4-2
ventilation 4-11
ventilation mechanics 4-12
ventilator 4-7–4-8
weaning 11-6
Assist/Control
pressure 3-12
graphics 5-17, 5-19
volume 3-6
graphics 5-16, 5-18
Asthma 9-11–9-15
acid-base 9-11
guidelines 9-14
invasive management 9-13
noninvasive support 9-12

pathophysiology 9-11
strategies 9-15
ASV. See Adaptive Support Ventilation (ASV)
Asynchrony 4-21, 7-44
cycle 7-50
expiratory valves 7-46
flow 5-49, 7-50
humidifiers 7-46
mode 7-49
rate 5-48
trigger 5-50, 7-47
ATC. See Automatic Tube Compensation (ATC)
Atelectasis 10-3
10-2
strategies 10-3
Atelectrauma 10-12
Automatic Tube Compensation (ATC) 3-39
Automode 3-40
Auto-PEEP 7-17, 10-4–10-7
asynchrony 7-45
clinical effects 10-5
Cstat changes 4-13
definition 10-4
graphics 5-51

identifying 10-5
measuring 10-6
strategies to reduce 10-7
treating 7-29
AVts. *See* Adaptive Support Ventilation (ASV)

B

Bag-Valve-Mask 7-2
Bariatrics 9-16–9-17
  invasive management 9-17
  noninvasive support 9-16
  pathophysiology 9-16
  weaning 9-17
Base Excess 6-2
Berlin definition, ARDS 9-3
Bias Flow (HFOV) 3-55
BiLevel. *See* Airway Pressure Release Ventilation (APRV)
Biotrauma 10-12
BiVent. *See* Airway Pressure Release Ventilation (APRV)
Blood Phase Symbols A-2

Blood Pressure
  mean 6-24
Body Surface Area 6-29
Bohr Equation 6-13
BP Fistula. *See* Bronchopleural Fistula
Breath Types 3-2
Bronchiectasis
  percussive therapies 7-41
Bronchopleural Fistula 9-18–9-19
  graphics 5-46
  invasive management 9-17
  management of 9-18
  weaning 9-19
Bronchospasm 4-4
Burns 7-17–7-18
  complications 9-20
  invasive management 9-20
  management of 9-20
  prophylactic support 1-2
  weaning 9-21

C

CABG. *See* Coronary Artery Bypass Graft

CaO_2 4-9, 4-10
Capnography
  Capography/Capnometry During Mechanical Ventilation A-7
  confirming ET tube placement 7-7
Capping Trials 7-14
Carbon Monoxide Poisoning 9-21
Cardiac
  acute event management 9-22
  effects of ventilation 10-16
  post-surgery management 9-24
Cardiac Output
  equation 6-23
  Fick Equation 6-24
Cardiogenic Pulmonary Edema. *See* Congestive Heart Failure
Cardiovascular
  acute respiratory failure 1-6
  weaning assessment 11-12
$C(a-v)O_2$ 4-10, 6-5
Central Nervous System Depression
  respiratory failure 1-5
Cerebral Contusion 9-38
Cerebral Perfusion Pressure 9-38
Chest

trauma 9-35
wiggle factor 3-55
Chest Imaging
  and weaning 11-11
Chest Wall Oscillations 7-39
Chronic Obstructive Pulmonary Disease 9-25–9-28
Cstat 4-13
  intrinsic PEEP 2-10
  invasive management 9-27
  management 9-28
  noninvasive support 9-26
  severity 9-25
  weaning 9-28
CO_2 Production 7-17
Compliance
  dynamic 4-12, 4-13
  equation 6-20
  static 4-12
    changes in 4-13
Congestive Heart Failure 9-22
  invasive management 9-23
  noninvasive support 9-22
Continuous Positive Airway Pressure
  invasive mode 3-38

noninvasive 8-4
Contusion. *See* Pulmonary Contusion
Conversions A-3
COPD. *See* Chronic Obstructive Pulmonary Disease
Coronary Artery Bypass Graft 9-24
Coronaviruses. *See* Viral Pulmonary Disorders
COVID. *See* Viral Pulmonary Disorders
CROP index 11-8
Cuff
  tracheostomy tube 7-10
  troubleshooting 4-4
Cuff Leak Test 11-20
  qualitative 11-20
  quantitative 11-20
Cuirass 7-39
CvO_2 4-10
Cycle
  asynchrony 7-50
  criteria 5-53
  time 2-26
  variable 3-2
Cylinders, Gas
  duration 6-30

D

Daily Sedation Interruption 11-2
Deadspace 7-17
  assessment 4-11
  to tidal volume ratio 1-8
  ventilation 6-12
  volume 6-13
Dead Space/Tidal Volume Ratio 6-13
Decannulation 7-14, 11-4
Delta-P. *See* Driving Pressure
  noninvasive 8-5
Derecruitment 10-3
  open lung approach 10-13
Difficult Airway 7-4
Difficult-to-Wean 11-4
Diffuse Axonal Injury 9-38
Discontinuation 11-4. *See also* Weaning
  Cardiovascular Assessment 11-12
  Definitions 11-4
  Electrolyte Assessment 11-12
  Metabolic Assessment 11-14
  Miscellaneous Factors 11-17
  Neurologic Assessment 11-14

Nutritional Assessment 11-13
Pharmacological Assessment 11-15
Renal Assessment 11-15
DO_2 6-8
Driving Pressure 2-14, 6-22, 9-4
   calculating 2-14
Drop and Stretch (APRV) 3-25
Drug Overdose 9-29–9-30
   invasive management 9-30
   monitoring 9-30
   noninvasive support 9-29
   weaning 9-30
Dynamic Compliance 4-12, 6-21
   equation 6-21
Dyssynchrony. See Asynchrony

E

ECMO. See Extracorporeal Membrane Oxygenation
Edi Catheter 3-44–3-45
Electrolytes
   weaning assessment 11-13
End-Expiratory Pause 10-6
Endotracheal Tube 7-4
   and auto-PEEP 10-7
   removal of (AARC CPG) A-11
   sizes 7-4
   suctioning (AARC CPG) A-8
   troubleshooting 4-4
EPAP 8-1, 8-5–8-7
Equations
   acid-base 6-2
   oxygenation 6-4
   patient calculations 6-29
   perfusion/hemodynamic 6-23
   ventilation 6-12
   ventilator calculations 6-16
Esophageal Detector Device 7-5
   verification 7-7
$ETCO_2$
   assessment 4-11
ET Tube. See Endotracheal Tube
Exchange ratio 6-11
Expiratory Hold 2-10, 2-19, 4-7
Expiratory Positive Airway Pressure 8-5, 8-5–8-7
Expiratory Time 2-19
   and auto-PEEP 2-10, 10-7
   and HFOV 3-55
   and I:E ratio 2-18
   and obstructive disorders 2-15
   calculating 2-19
Expiratory Trigger 2-21
Expiratory Valves
   and auto-PEEP 10-7
   asynchrony 7-46
Extracorporeal Membrane Oxygenation 3-51–3-53
   ARDS 9-5
   types 3-52
   ventilator settings 3-53
   weaning 3-53
Extrapulmonary Effects 10-16
Extubation 11-4
   and cuff leak test 11-20
   post-extubation care 11-21
   procedure 11-21
   Removal of the Endotracheal Tube A-11, A-12
   stridor 11-22

F

FEV1 1-8
Fick Equation 6-24
Fighting the Ventilator. *See* Asynchrony
FIO_2 2-4, 2-20, 7-23
   average 2-20
   calculating 7-23
   calculating new 2-20
   error 4-20
   estimation 6-6
   oxygenation 7-23
Flail Chest 9-35
Flow Asynchrony 5-49, 7-50
Flow Starvation 5-49
Flow-Time Scalar 5-9
   applications 5-10
Flow-Volume Loop 5-14
   applications 5-15
Flow Waveform
   types 2-4
Fractures, Rib 9-35
FRC. *See* Functional Residual Capacity (FRC)
Frequency. *See* Rate
Functional Lung Size 6-22
Functional Residual Capacity (FRC) 2-10
   clinical parameter 1-8
f/Vt. *See* Rapid Shallow Breathing Index

G

Gag Reflex 11-10
Gas Phase Symbols A-2
Gas Supply
   calculating 6-30
   troubleshooting 4-20
Gastric
   effects of ventilation 10-17
Granulation Tissue 7-11
Graphics. *See* Ventilator Graphics
Guillain Barré Syndrome. *See* Neuromuscular Disorders

H

HCO_3^-
   estimation 6-3
Head Injury. *See also* Trauma (Head)
   prophylactic support 1-2
Heat and Moisture Exchanger
   resistance 4-8
Height
   calculating tidal volume 2-7
   conversion table A-4
Hemodynamic Monitoring
   equations 6-23
Hemothorax 1-5
Henderson-Hasselbach 6-3
Hepatic
   effects of ventilation 10-17
Hertz 3-55
High-Flow Nasal Cannula 8-2
High-Flow Oxygen Therapy 8-2
   settings 8-3
   weaning 8-3
High Frequency Chest Wall Oscillation (HFCWO) 7-39
High-Frequency Oscillatory Ventilation (HFOV) 3-54
   ARDS 9-5
   clinical notes 3-59
   definitions 3-55
   managing 3-58

settings 3-56
troubleshooting 3-60–3-61
weaning 3-59
HME. *See* Heat and Moisture Exchanger
Horowitz Index 6-10
Humidification 2-22, 7-42
   AARC guideline 7-43, A-9
   and NIV 8-3
   asynchrony 7-46, 10-11
   excess 7-11
   goals of 2-22
   heated 7-43
   insufficient 7-11
   types of 2-22
Hypercapnia
   permissive 7-20, 9-4
Hyperoxic Lung Injury 10-8
   strategies 10-8
Hyperventilation 4-11, 10-15
   and brain injury 9-40
   respiratory alkalosis 11-9
Hypoventilaton 10-14
Hypoxemia 2-20
   and lung injury 10-12
   permissive 10-13
   refractory 7-32, 9-3, 10-10
Hypoxemic Respiratory Failure 1-4. *See also* Viral Pulmonary Disorders
Hypoxia
   assessing (equation) 6-4

I

Ideal Body Weight (IBW) 2-7, 6-29
I:E Ratio 2-4, 2-18
   alarm 2-23
   and inspiratory time 2-16
   and rate 2-15
   inverse 7-36
   relationship 2-26
InCourage 7-39
Independent Lung Ventilation (ILV) 9-43
   procedure 9-43
   settings 9-43
Indirect Calorimetry 6-11
Infection 10-18
Inflection Points 5-45
Initiation 8-4
   checklist 1-10

Inspiratory:Expiratory Ratio. *See* I: E Ratio
Inspiratory Hold 2-8
   measure of Pplat 2-13
Inspiratory Pause 2-16
Inspiratory Positive Airway Pressure (IPAP) 8-5
Inspiratory Time 2-4, 2-16
   average 2-16
   cautions 2-16
   definition 2-16
   graphics 5-54
Inspiratory Trigger. *See* Trigger
Intracerebral Hemorrhage 9-38
Intracranial Pressure 9-38, 9-41
   and hyperventilation 9-41
   management 9-41
   symptoms 9-41
Intrapulmonary Percussive Ventilation (IPV) 7-40
Intraventricular Hemorrhage 9-38
Intubation 7-5
   confirmation 7-6
   equipment 7-5
   procedure 7-5
Inverse Ratio Ventilation (IRV) 7-36

IPAP. *See* Inspiratory Positive Airway Pressure

K

Kyphoscoliosis 1-5
   Cstat 4-13
Kyphosis 1-5

L

Laryngoscope 7-5
Leak
   assessing 4-16, 4-18
   cuff 4-4
   graphics 5-46
   troubleshooting 4-18
   ventilator 4-5
Left Ventricular Stroke Work
   equation 6-24
Liberation 11-4. *See also* Weaning
Loops. *See* Ventilator Graphics
Lung Abscess. *See* Unilateral Disorders
Lung Distension
   compliance equation 6-20
Lung Injury 10-12
   damage cascade 10-13
   hyperoxic 10-8
   objectives 1-9
Lung Protective Strategies 10-13
   permissive hypercapnia 7-20
   permissive hypoxemia 10-13
Lung Transplantation. *See* Unilateral Disorders
LVSW 6-24

M

Mallampati Score 7-4
Mandatory Minute Ventubation (MMV)
   pressure 3-18
   volume 3-10
MAP. *See* Mean Airway Pressure; *See* Mean Arterial Blood Pressure
Maximal Inspiratory Pressure. *See* PIMax
Mean Airway Pressure 2-4, 2-12, 7-32
   average 2-12
   calculating 7-32
   calculation 2-12
   definition 2-12
   determinants 2-28
   equation 6-22
   oxygenation 7-32
Mean Arterial Pressure 6-24
Mean Pulmonary Artery Pressure 6-25
Metabolic 11-9
   acidosis 7-19
   alkalosis 7-19
   assessment 11-13
   disorders 7-19
   weaning assessment 11-13
MetaNeb 7-39
Metric Conversions A-3
Minute Ventilation 2-4, 2-5, 6-14, 7-15
   and auto-PEEP 10-7
   and reintubation 11-23
   assessment 4-11
   calculations 2-5
   nomogram 6-14
   relationships 2-25
   ventilator estimate 7-15
MMV. *See* Mandatory Minute Ventilation (MMV)
Mode Asynchrony 7-49
Modes of Ventilation
   breath types 3-2
   chart of 3-3
   classification 3-2

key 3-4
selecting 3-1
Morbid Obesity. *See* Bariatrics
mPAW. *See* Mean Airway Pressure;
See Mean Arterial Pressure
Myasthenia Gravis 9-31
Myocardial Infarction (MI)
 invasive management 9-23
 management of 9-23
 noninvasive support 9-22

N

Nasal Trumpet 7-3
Nasopharyngeal Airway 7-3
National Asthma Education Guidelines 9-13
Neurally Adjusted Ventilatory Assist (NAVA)
 3-41–3-50
 Edi catheter 3-44
 explanation 3-42
 indications 3-43
 risks 3-43
 selection algorithm 3-47
 settings (invasive) 3-46
 settings (noninvasive) 3-48
 troubleshooting 3-49–3-50
Neurologic
 effects of ventilation 10-16
 weaning assessment 11-14
Neuromuscular Disorders 9-31–9-32
 acute respiratory failure 1-6
 invasive management 9-32
 management 9-32
 respiratory parameters 9-31
 weaning 9-32
NIV. *See* Noninvasive Ventilation
NIV-NAVA. *See* Neurally Adjusted Ventilatory Assist (NAVA)
Noncardiogenic Pulmonary Edema.
 See Congestive Heart Failure
Noninvasive Continuous Positive Airway
 Pressure (CPAP) 8-4
Noninvasive Positive Pressure Ventilation
 (NPPV) 8-5
 indications 8-5
 initiation 8-5
 management 8-6
 settings 8-6
Noninvasive Ventilation (NIV) 8-1–8-12
 assessment of improvement 8-9
 complications 8-11
 considerations 8-11
 contraindications 8-9
 CPAP 8-4
 failure (discontinuing) 8-12
 interfaces (masks) 8-10
 management (ARF) 8-8
 monitoring 8-12
 NPPV (BiPAP) 8-5
 terminology 8-1
NPPV. *See* Noninvasive Positive Pressure
 Ventilation (NPPV)
Nutrition
 effects of ventilation 10-17

O

O_2. *See* Oxygen
O_2 Extraction Ratio 6-8
Obesity. *See* Bariatrics
Obstruction
 airway 1-5, 10-2
 airway resistance 4-14

graphics 5-44
Obstructive Disorders
  rate setting 2-15
Obstructive Sleep Apnea 1-5
OI. See Oxygen Index
Open Lung Approach 10-13
Oropharyngeal Airway 7-3
OSA. See Obstructive Sleep Apnea
Oscillatory PEP Therapy 7-39
Overdistension 7-32
  and PEEP level 7-25
  graphics 5-45
  volutrauma 10-12
Oxygen. See also FIO2
  amount (equation) 6-7
  content 4-10
  extraction ratio 4-10
  index 4-10
  partial pressure 1-8, 4-10
  P/F ratio 4-10
  S/F ratio 4-10
Oxygenation
  and mPAW 2-12
  assessing 4-10, 7-30
  determinants 2-28
  estimate 7-21
  improving 7-21–7-35
  weaning assessment 11-7
Oxygen Consumption 6-6
  tissues 6-5, 6-6
Oxygen Content 4-9, 6-7
  arterial 6-7
  mixed venous 6-7
  pulmonary capillary 6-7
Oxygen Delivery 6-8
Oxygen Index 6-9, 7-21
Oxygen Percentage. See Oxygen
Oxygen Reserve 6-9
Oxygen Saturation 6-9, 6-10
Oxygen Toxicity. See Hyperoxic Lung Injury

P

P0.1 4-12, 11-8
PaCO$_2$ 1-8
  assessment 4-11
  estimation 6-3
Palv 2-13
PaO$_2$ 1-8, 4-10
  predicted 6-11
PAO$_2$ 6-4
PaO$_2$/FIO$_2$. See P/F Ratio
Parameters 2-4
  weaning 11-2
Patient Assessment 4-6
Patient Positioning 7-33
  proning 7-33
Patient-Ventilator Asynchrony. See Asynchrony
PAV. See Proportional Assist Ventilation (PAV)
PBW 6-29. See Predicted Body Weight
Peak Inspiratory Pressure 2-4
  average 2-9
  definition 2-9
Pectus Deformities 1-5
  carinatum 1-5
  excavatum 1-5
Pectus Excavatum
  Cstat 4-13
PEEP 7-24. See Positive End Expiratory Pressure; See also Oxygen
  Applied 7-29
  Ranges 7-25

treating auto-PEEP 7-29
PEEP-compensated 3-12
Percussionator 7-39
PercussiveNeb 7-39
Percussive Vests/Wraps 7-41
Permissive Hypercapnia 7-20, 7-21, 9-4, 10-13
   and auto-PEEP 10-7
Permissive Hypoxemia 10-13
P/F Ratio 1-8, 4-10, 6-10, 7-21
   assessing PEEP 7-30
pH 1-8
Physiological VD/VT Ratio 6-13
PImax 4-12
   clinical parameter 1-8
PIP. See Peak Inspiratory Pressure
Plateau Pressure 2-13
   average 2-13
   definition 2-13
   graphics 5-52
   measuring auto-PEEP 10-6
Pleural Disease 1-5
Pneumonia. See Unilateral Disorders
Pneumothorax 9-35
   acute respiratory failure 1-5

   contraindication to PPV 1-3
Poisoning. See Drug Overdose
Positioning, Patient 7-33
   oxygenation 7-33
   unilateral disorders 9-42
Positive End Expiratory Pressure 2-4. See also Auto-PEEP
   and P-V loop 7-27
   assessing 7-30
   by chest radiograph 7-28
   by P/F ratio 7-28
   changes in 4-19
   definition 2-10
   extrinsic 2-10
   for auto-PEEP 7-29
   initiation 7-25
   intrinsic 2-10
   monitoring 2-11
   optimal 2-11, 7-26
   oxygenation 7-24
   ranges 7-25
   tables (ARDSnet) 9-8
   weaning 7-31
Post-Extubation Care 11-20
Postoperative Management 9-33

   Management of 9-34, 9-42
Post-Perfusion Injury 9-2
Post Polio Syndrome. See Neuromuscular Disorders
Post-Resuscitation Hypoxia 9-38
Predicted Body Weight 2-7, 6-29
Predicted PaO₂ 6-11
Pressure
   driving 2-8, 2-14, 6-22
   mean airway 2-12
   peak inspiratory 2-9
   plateau 2-13
Pressure-Regulated Volume Control 3-29
Pressure Support 3-16
   graphics 5-17, 5-19
Pressure-Time Scalar 5-4
   applications 5-6
Pressure Ventilation
   graphics 5-17, 5-19
   modes chart 3-3
   operating relationships 2-27
Pressure Ventilation (Modes) 3-3
   APRV 3-20
   APV 3-31
   Assist/Control 3-12

ASV 3-37
BiLevel 3-20
BiVent 3-20
CPAP 3-38
MMV 3-18
PAV 3-32
PPS 3-32
PRVC 3-29
PSV 3-16
SIMV 3-14
SmartCare PS 3-34
TCAV 3-20
VAPS 3-26
VS 3-35
Pressure-Volume Loop 5-11
 applications 5-13
Proning 7-33
 artificial airway 7-35
 management 7-35
 procedure 7-34
Prophylactic Ventilatory Support 1-2
Proportional Assist Ventilation (PAV) 3-32
Proportional Pressure Support 3-32
PRVC. *See* Pressure-Regulated Volume Control

Pulmonary Artery Pressure
 mean 6-25
Pulmonary Contusion 9-35
Pulmonary Edema
 cardiogenic 9-22
 noncardiogenic 9-2
Pulmonary Embolus 7-17
Pulmonary Vascular Resistance 6-25
Pulmonary Vasodilators
 and ARDS 9-5
Pulse Oximetry
 clinical range 4-10
Pulse Pressure 6-26
P-V Loop
 PEEP setting 7-27
PvO_2 4-10
PVR 6-25

Q

QT 6-23

R

Rapid Shallow Breathing Index 6-18, 11-19
 considerations 11-19
 performing 11-19
 signs of failure 11-18
Rate 2-4, 2-15
 asynchrony 5-48
 average 2-15
 calculating 2-15
 changes in 4-17
 definition 2-15
 relationships 2-26
 ventilator estimate 7-15
RE 6-11
Refractory Hypoxemia
 oxygen index 6-9
Reintubation 11-23
Renal
 effects of ventilation 10-17
Respiratory
 distress 4-2
 drive 4-12, 10-9
 muscle strength 4-12

Respiratory Acidosis
  ventilator strategies 7-16
Respiratory Alkalosis 4-11
  ventilator strategies 7-18
Respiratory Distress
  assessing 4-6
Respiratory Failure
  checklist 1-5
  chronic 1-2
  impending 1-2
  type I 1-4
  type II 1-4
Respiratory Index 6-11
Respiratory Quotient 6-11
Restrictive Disorders 9-34
RI 6-11
Right Ventricular Stroke Work 6-26
Rise Time
  graphics 5-53
RSBI 4-12, 6-18. *See* Rapid Shallow Breathing Index
Rule of 8's 6-3
RVSW 6-26

S

SaO2 1-8, 4-10, 6-10
  saturation 4-10
SBT. *See* Spontaneous Breathing Trial
Scalars 5-4
  pressure-time 5-5
  volume-time 5-7
Secretions
  causing Raw 4-14
Sedation
  daily interruption 11-2
Sensitivity 2-21, 7-47, 7-48
Sepsis 7-17
  and ARDS 9-2
Settings 8-4
S/F ratio 4-10, 7-21
Shock
  prophylactic support 1-2
Shunt
  equation 6-27
Shunt Equation 6-27
Simplified Weaning Index 11-8
SIMV. *See* Synchronized Intermittent Mandatory Ventilation (SIMV)
Skin Integrity
  and proning 7-35
Sleep Disordered Breathing
  acute respiratory failure 1-5
SmartCare Pressure Support 3-34
SmartVest 7-39
Smoke Inhalation. *See* Burns
Speaking Valves 7-9
SpO2 4-10
Spontaneous Breathing Trial 11-4
  definition 11-4
Spontaneous Ventilation
  graphics 5-16
Stroke (CVA) 9-38
Stroke Volume 6-28
Subarachnoid Hemorrhage 9-38
Subdural Hematoma 9-38
Subglottic Tubes 7-4
Suctioning 7-37
  catheter size formula 7-38
  indications 7-37
  pressures 7-38
Surgical
  prophylactic support 1-2

SV 6-28
SvO₂ 4-10, 6-9
SVR 6-28
Synchronized Intermittent Mandatory Ventilation (SIMV)
   pressure 3-14
   volume 3-4, 3-8
Synchrony 7-44–7-49
   assessing 4-8
Systemic Vascular Resistance 6-28

T

TCAV. *See* Airway Pressure Release Ventilation (APRV)
TCO₂ 4-9
Temperature
   conversion table A-4
Tension Pneumothorax 4-4
TI. *See* Inspiratory Time
Tidal Volume (VT) 2-4, 2-6
   calculating 2-7
   changes in 4-16
   clinical parameter 1-8
   relationships 2-25
   ventilator estimate 7-15
Time
   expiratory 2-19
   inspiratory 2-16
Time Constant 2-16, 6-23
Time-Controlled Adaptive Ventilation. *See* Airway Pressure Release Ventilation (APRV)
T-Piece Adapter
   measuring auto-PEEP 10-6
Tracheostomy 7-8
   care 7-9, 7-12
   changing 7-12
   considerations 7-13
   troubleshooting 4-4, 7-10
Transfusions
   and ARDS 9-2
Transport (intra-hospital) (AARC CPG) A-10
Trauma
   and ARDS 9-2
   prophylactic support 1-2
Trauma (Chest) 9-35–9-37
   blunt 9-35
   flail segment 9-35
   invasive management 9-36
   management of 9-34, 9-42
   noninvasive support 9-36
   penetrating 9-35
   weaning 9-37
Trauma (Head) 9-38–9-41
   guidelines 9-40
   invasive management 9-38
   monitoring CPP and ICP 9-38, 9-41
   weaning 9-41
Trigger 2-21
   asynchrony 5-50, 7-47
   average 2-21
   definition 2-21
   graphics 5-16
Troubleshooting
   patient 4-4
   ventilator 4-5, 4-15–4-21

U

Unilateral Disorders 9-42
U.S. Customary Conversions A-3

V

VA 6-12
V-A/C. *See* Assist-Control
VAE. *See* Ventilator Injury
VAE ECMO 3-52
VAP. *See* Ventilator Injury
 VAE Bundle 10-20
VAPS. *See* Volume-Assured Pressure Support
VC. *See* Vital Capacity
V_D 6-12
V_{Dphys} 4-11
V_D/V_T 1-8, 4-11, 6-13
V_E 6-14. *See* Minute Ventilation
Venoarterial ECMO 3-52
Venous Blood Gas
 values 4-9
Venovenous ECMO 3-52
Ventilation
 assessment 4-11
 mechanics 4-12
Ventilation/Perfusion 6-15
 imbalances 10-10
 strategies to improve 10-10
Ventilator
 and proning 7-35
 assessment 4-7
 calculations 6-16
 circuit
  assessing 4-8
  extrapulmonary effects 10-16
  infections 10-18
  leak 4-5
 malfunction 4-2
 obstructions 4-5
 power loss 4-20
 pressures 2-8
 pulmonary effects 10-2
Ventilator Associated Events 10-19
Ventilator Graphics
 explanations 5-3
 indications 5-3
 loops 5-11
 normal 5-16-5-25
 scalars 5-4-5-10
 types 5-4
Ventilator Injury 10-12
Ventilatory Drive
 and weaning 11-11
 Factors increasing or decreasing 11-11
Ventilatory Support
 contraindications 1-3
 full vs. partial 2-2
 indications 1-2
 initiation 1-10
 objectives 1-9
  clinical 1-9
  physiological 1-9
  volume vs. pressure 2-3
Vest Therapy 7-41
Viral Pulmonary Disorders 9-44-9-46
 invasive management 9-45
 management 9-45
 noninvasive support 9-44
 weaning 9-46
Vital Capacity 4-12
 clinical parameter 1-8
Vital Signs
 weaning assessment 11-6
VO_2 6-6, 6-24
Volume - Assist/Control. *See* Assist/Control
Volume-Assured Pressure Support 3-26

Volume Support 3-35
Volume-Time Scalar 5-7
   applications 5-8
Volume Ventilation
   graphics 5-16, 5-18
   mode chart 3-3
   operating relationships 2-24
Volume Ventilation (Modes) 3-3
   Assist/Control 3-6
   MMV 3-10
   SIMV 3-8
Volutrauma 10-12
VQI 4-10
$\dot{V}/\dot{Q}$ Ratio 6-15
VS. *See* Volume Support
Vt. *See* Tidal Volume
VV ECMO 3-52

   assessments 11-6, 11-6–11-16
   discontinuation assessment 11-3
   Failure 11-18
   guidelines 11-24
   parameters 11-2
   predictive indices 11-7
   procedures 11-17
   prolonged 11-4
   strategies 11-5
   terminology 11-4
Weight
   conversion table A-4
White-Out (CXR) 9-4
Winters' Formula 6-3
Work of Breathing (WOB) 10-11
   assessment 10-11
   causes 10-11
   strategies to improve 10-11

W

Waveform Graphics. *See* Ventilator Graphics
Weaning. *See also* Discontinuation
   algorithm 11-2
   and lung protection 10-13